Warrior Women

Warrior Women
Reshni Ratnam

Design and Layout: Preston Jongbloed.
www.brandgrowth.co.za
preston@brandgrowth.co.za
0768818479

ISBN: 9780646826967

CONTENTS

CONTENTS

Acknowledgements

This book would not have been made possible had I not given birth to my two beautiful premature babies – Isla May Ratnam-Elmore and Rohaan Harry David Ratnam-Elmore.

My children have made me stronger than I could imagine and more determined than ever to normalise the struggles of pregnancy and birth.

To the sisterhood, thank you for sharing your stories with me, and with the world. Thank you for being open, honest and disclosing the hardest times in your lives.

My heartfelt thanks to neonatologist Dr Luke Jardine at Brisbane's Mater Mothers' Hospital, and to the Royal Brisbane and Women's Hospital's neonatology director and Queensland Milk Bank director Dr Pieter Koorts, for taking the time to share their expertise and words of wisdom.

My dreams of becoming a parent are now a reality thanks to general practitioner Dr Su-Min Khoo, obstetrician Dr Alex Alexander and my children's paediatrician Dr Aaron Easterbrook.

You have been there for me through the good times and the bad.

And lastly, a special thanks to my husband Craig Elmore, the love of my life, for encouraging me to write this book. I have wanted to fulfil this dream since 2017 – the year I became a mum of a premature baby.

Thank you for making this happen.

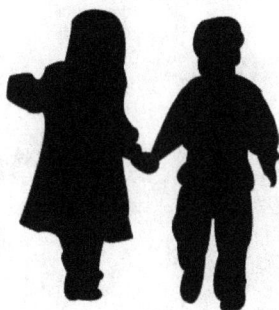

1

Twice unexpected

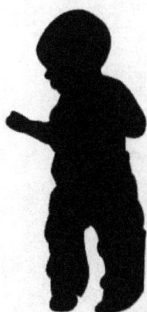

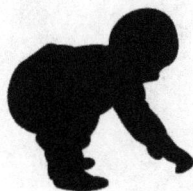

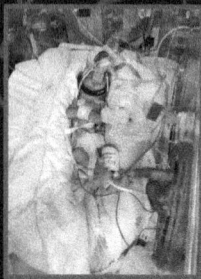

Isla was born on November 3, 2017, weighing 1200g

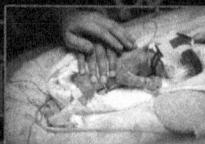

Isla spent about eight weeks in the NICCU.
Photo: Ric Frearson

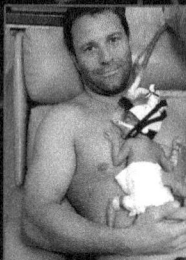

Craig's first cuddle with Isla.

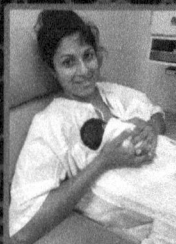

Isla was so tiny and fragile. I looked forward to my daily cuddles with her.

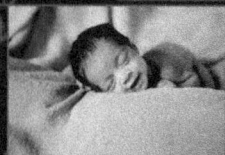

After two months in hospital we finally got to bring Isla home.
Photo: Ric Frearson

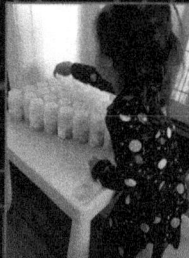

Isla now helps count my milk stash which is donated to the Qld Milk Bank.

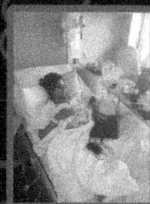

While on two weeks bedrest I continued to work from the hospital, helping to take my mind off things.

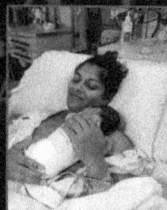

I had my first cuddle with Rohaan severa hours after he w born.

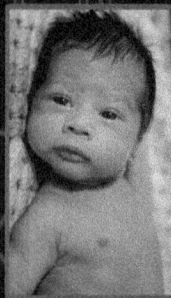

Rohaan was born at 34+1 weeks' after my waters broke unexpectedly.

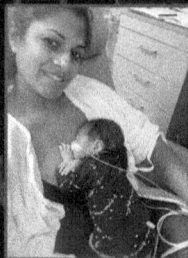

Rohaan gained weight quickly while in hospital for two weeks.

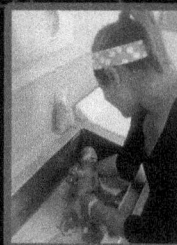

Rohaan's first bath.

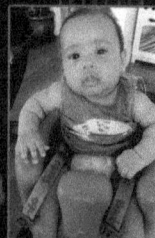

Rohaan the mil monster at thre months of age.

Experiencing motherhood is a dream come true. There are highs, and some days there are lows, but I am forever grateful that I am able to hold my two babies in my arms at night and tuck them into bed.

As a young girl, I always wanted to be a mother — to nurture and care for children of my own. After giving birth to two premature babies, I know all too well what having a 'miracle baby' is about. In fact, all babies are beautiful little miracles. Everyone has a birth story and every story is so different. My daughter Isla was born at 29+1 weeks' gestation. I had a fall at work and she was delivered via an emergency caesarean (c-section) at Brisbane's Mater Mothers' Hospital the very next day. I am ever so thankful to my obstetrician Dr Alex Alexander, general practitioner Dr Su-Min Khoo and the kids' paediatrician Dr Aaron Easterbrook. These Brisbane medical professionals have played a vital role in seeing my dreams come true.

Isla was born on November 3, 2017. My husband and I were thrown into parenthood in an instant. Our nursery wasn't ready and I'd only just figured out where the brake was on the pram that week. I was very much looking forward to my baby shower... and having some time off work prior to the birth. We knew we were having a little girl and had her name picked out. My husband loved the name Isla and claimed naming rights when we started dating.

Throughout my pregnancy I remained fit and active.I walked our rescue dog Maple every day, enjoyed light exercise at the gym and continued my Saturday morning Park Run ritual (at a slower pace). So when I fell over at work unexpectedly, I was taken by surprise.

The day after I fell, in the early hours of the morning, I texted my friend Louise and told her what had happened. I had also just experienced a very light mucus-type bleed. At the time Louise was tending to her newborn and advised me to call the hospital pronto, and book in to see my obstetrician. Boy, am I glad I did.

Being so engrossed in my work as a journalist, I didn't think much of the fall. Craig and I had our antenatal classes booked, but sadly never had the chance to attend. I didn't know how serious a fall was during pregnancy, until the day my daughter arrived. I was monitored in hospital for several hours after seeing Dr Alexander that morning. Nurses came and went. They called Dr Alexander and kept him updated on the baby's heart rate. I have a high pain threshold, so didn't think much of the cramps in my tummy overnight. But I later found out they were contractions.

After being taken for my second scan of the day, I was told I was 2cm dilated. The baby's heart rate was deceleratingand her chances of surviving meant she had to be born quickly. Dr Alexander came to my bedside after speaking with one of the nurses on duty. I asked him if I could go home and pack some clothes and get a few things ready. He said "Reshni, we have 10 minutes to get this baby out, we are heading to theatre now". Tears streamed from my eyes, I couldn't believe my baby would be born 11 weeks early. I had failed my daughter. I couldn't even carry her full term.

I often think back to the day I had the fall at work. It was flat ground. I didn't trip over anything. I didn't fall down a flight of stairs. It all happened so quickly.

Why did it happen? Was the fall the cause of my pre-term baby? Or was she just ready to see the world, and the fall was a message to say 'I'm on my way'. No one can explain it. It's one of those things.

As I was overcome with guilt, my husband had turned pale and crouched next to my bed. "Wow, I'm not sure I'm ready for this," he said."I feel faint". So the nurses tended to Craig and told him to wash his face with water, and quickly get into his scrubs. As they wheeled me to theatre I heard the doctors and nurses pandering over Craig, asking if he was okay and if he needed to sip on some juice. I was thinking "Ummmm, hello! Don't worry about him, what about me?" Craig was asked to remain outside the theatre room until I had my epidural administered. I guess no one wants to deal with a father fainting during an emergency c-section, do they? So when he finished powdering his nose (no, I mean getting ready for the momentous arrival of our first child), I looked at him (more like rolling my eyes) and said "you've got one job" and that's to take photos or find someone to take them'. And let me tell you, he took the best photos of our beautiful little girl being born. Luckily (for Craig) he recovered after the initial moments of shock subsided. He went from nearly fainting to being 'up close and personal' watching our baby being born.

The sixth floor at Brisbane's Mater Mothers' Hospital practically became my home as our fragile baby tried to gain weight. As the days passed, reality set in. I was sad. I blamed myself for months. If I hadn't fallen over would Isla have had this start to life?

I became familiar with the nurses and they guided me through looking after a premature baby. Some days I sobbed uncontrollably, holding my tender c-section wound, watching my daughter's every movement in her incubator.

For eight weeks I visited my little girl in the hospital. I pumped milk around the clock to give her what she needed. I sat in front of her incubator every morning and every night. I stared at the cord-heavy white walls surrounding her incubator and tried to make sense of the monitors and their various sounds. I held her NG tube (Nasogastric tube used for infants and children who are not able to take in enough calories by mouth) so she could ingest my expressed milk. I remember the immense relief I felt when she could tolerate a measly 3ml at a time and got excited when her feeds increased from 5ml to 10ml. It wasn't long until I started meeting the other mothers coming and going from their rooms.

Every day I prayed Isla would survive and make it through another night. My friends and family rallied around us and helped deliver my expressed milk to the hospital every day. I couldn't drive for several weeks and I am forever touched by their generosity, with someone always making sure I could be by Isla's side in the hospital. They brought us meals so we were well fed, and sent messages of support. My friends sat around my bedside hours after I gave birth and gave me the support and the encouragement I needed. They came to my house while my baby was in hospital and said "mumma, you got this". This is what I needed to hear.

My parents were emotionally fragile. My mum was broken, she had been overseas when Isla unexpectedly decided to make her entrance into the world. She had tears every time she came to the hospital. She struggled with the constant beeping of monitors and seeing her granddaughter with a nasal feeding tube.

But my mum and dad prayed every day for our daughter to come home well and healthy. My mother-in-law and father-in-law were sad for us, but happy our baby girl had showed signs of progress ever so quickly. My mother-in-law's knitting group banded together to sew some beautiful beanies and booties for our pint-size princess. Friends at her local church checked in to see how we were coping. It was very touching.

While my husband and I were dealing with the stress of having a premature baby in hospital, so too were our parents. I knew I had to be strong for not only my daughter, but those around us. I didn't want to show them any signs of weakness. I cried in the shower and I cried into my pillow at night. I was sad for the babies coming into the NICU, but happy they too were given a second chance. I was jealous when other babies got to go home before mine did. But eventually our day came. After two months in hospital, we brought Isla home on Christmas Eve, 2017. Another extra special day on our calendar now.

And then... Come 2020, during the height of a global pandemic (COVID-19) our son Rohaan was born. Another little miracle was welcomed into our family. People assume that after having one premature baby things are a lot easier the second time around.

I had been on a high dose of drugs to keep my baby in longer this time. It was picked up during one of my scans that I had placenta previa (low lying placenta). Placenta previa occurs when a baby's placenta partially or totally covers the mother's cervix — the outlet for the uterus. It can cause severe bleeding during pregnancy and delivery. So a vaginal birth was not on the cards during what was deemed a high-risk pregnancy.

One night after taking a shower, my waters broke unexpectedly at 32 weeks' gestation. It was a very, very light trickle of amniotic fluid. Not the 'big gush' everyone talks about. My gut instinct was to call the Mater Mothers' Pregnancy Assessment Centre immediately and head straight in to be monitored. I wasn't taking any chances this time around. I drove myself to hospital that night for what I thought would be a quick check up and reassurance everything would be okay. Little did I know, I wasn't coming home until our baby was born.

I was on bedrest for two weeks at the Mater Mothers' Hospital in Brisbane. During the pandemic, the hospital only allowed the patient's main carer to visit (my husband), and no children were allowed. I was scared. I was lonely. I had let my family down again. The risk of infection was high and my obstetrician took no chances. Being on hospital bedrest also meant there was some hope of replenishing the lost amniotic fluid.

Two weeks dragged on and sadly I couldn't see my baby girl Isla, give her kisses and cuddles after childcare, or tuck her into bed at night. Prior to my waters breaking no plan was in place in the event I had another premature baby—everything had been tracking so well.

When I texted my husband to say I wasn't coming home until our baby boy arrived, we had to swiftly organise what to do if I went into labour. Thankfully my in-laws were on hand to help out with childcare drop-offs and pickups as my husband continued to work and juggle visits to the hospital. Some days he worked from the hospital too.

In a bid to save my sanity while in hospital, I indulged in peanut butter cheesecake and binged on Netflix shows. I also continued to file stories from my bedside for The Courier-Mail and The Sunday Mail, keeping in touch with my boss daily.

That helped take my mind off worrying if my unborn baby would be OK. 'The baby's still in there. We've made it through another day' I would text my friends and colleagues.

Daily injections and medication to stop the contractions, constant monitoring of the baby's heart rate and progesterone pessaries up my bum to keep the baby in was all in a day's work. Wondering why I had backdoor pessaries? Well, anything up your hoo-ha during the 'waiting game' is not recommended due to infection. I laid in hospital alone, nurses coming in to check on me every few hours. Even throughout the night I was woken to take certain medications at specific times. I hardly slept. I was busy joining super massive maternity pads together to catch the amniotic fluid which leaked and leaked and leaked, throughout the night. I would often have to call a nurse asking for extra maternity pads, new gowns and a change of bedsheets. It wasn't pleasant. But the hospital was the safest place for me to be.

Not having friends or family visit during my stay in hospital was difficult. I felt very isolated. I developed a cold and was told a COVID test was mandatory. So in came a lady all kitted up from head to toe to shove something up my nose and down my throat to make sure I wasn't infected with this disease which was killing people around the world.

Two weeks passed, then one Sunday morning on May 10, 2020 the pains became intense and I knew things were going to happen very quickly. Unfortunately, Dr Alexander was not rostered on that weekend and another obstetrician delivered our son. After hours of enduring severe labour pains, I called my husband at 5.30am and asked him to make his way to the hospital. "Can you ask your mum to babysit Isla for the day," I asked. I must have spoken ever so calmly, because when Craig arrived he was ready to set up his laptop and do some work from the hospital that morning.

"Oh, you won't have time for that today, we are having the baby now. We are waiting for you to get into your scrubs. I'm ready to go", I smiled.

Craig looked at me with wide eyes. "What, we're having the baby? Now?" he asked. "Yeah, I didn't want to panic you when I called. I thought calling at 5.30am telling you I was having contractions meant you would realise I was in labour," I said. Craig got dressed in his scrubs and I was wheeled downstairs to theatre.

Again tears streamed from my eyes. I had flashbacks to when my daughter was born. Another full term pregnancy was not achieved. I failed again. Rohaan was born at 34+1 weeks' gestation, weighing 2100g.

I heard him cry and it made me cry. It was Mother's Day and what a memorable day it will be for our family every year.

Rohaan was whisked away to NICU and my husband went with him. I knew he was bigger, older and stronger than his sister was when she was born, so I was calm knowing his time in hospital would be less. I couldn't wait to see him. To touch him. To smell him. And the moment I saw him in his incubator, I cried again. I had my first cuddle with my son that day. Unlike his sister, I had to wait three days before I could hold Isla. She was tiny and I didn't know what to do with her. She was ever so fragile.

Rohaan was ready to breastfeed and I couldn't wipe the smile off my face. It took Isla months to get the hang of breastfeeding. Some mums will tell you breastfeeding is easy, but that isn't the case for everyone. Not everyone can just "flop it out" and have their baby latch on like a legend. So, back to pumping every two hours, religiously setting the alarm on my phone to wake up.

Because if you've ever slept through a dedicated pumping session, you'll know about it. Massive leaking boobs and milk wasted. The nurses were ever so helpful, taking my expressed breastmilk downstairs to my son so he could be fed every two to three hours. Rohaan drank every millilitre of milk I produced and I had to pump more frequently to boost my supply.

After spending three weeks in hospital in total, I was keen to get home. I couldn't take Rohaan with me, yet. But like his sister, he too was a fighter. He stayed in for another two weeks.

My husband and I dropped milk off morning and night so he could gain weight and reach his milestones. And we even brought him home before his due date. Sadly, some parents don't get to take their babies home due to illness or ongoing medical problems.

While I did not require donated human milk for my son, I was able to donate several litres to the Queensland Milk Bank at the Royal Brisbane and Women's Hospital after Isla was born, and I have continued to do so with Rohaan. I remember the Mater nurses frequently telling me I was filling their fridge and freezers with my milk and they were running out of space. Both times upon discharge I was told to bring an esky to pack all my milk in to take home. The eskies we brought were so full and I decided to leave some milk behind so it could be donated to the Milk Bank (after going through all the required checks). Did you know breast milk increases the survival rate of premature babies by up to 70 per cent?

If it wasn't for Isla I would not have known about the Milk Bank. Human donor milk is easily digested and empties into the stomach faster than formula. Donating my milk is my way of giving back and helping other sick and preterm babies. Other than my time to express a little extra milk here and there, it doesn't cost me anything. So if you're anything like me - massive hooters and an endless supply of 'liquid gold' – then think about becoming a human milk donor.

The Queensland Milk Bank is ever so important and if I can encourage more mothers to donate milk to help sick and premature babies across Australia, then I know sharing my story has been worthwhile.

- Reshni Ratnam, proud mum to two premature babies

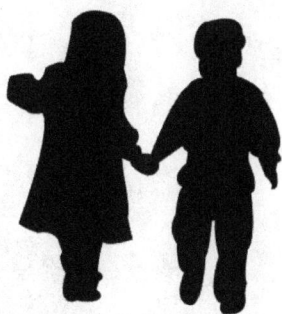

2

A miracle abroad

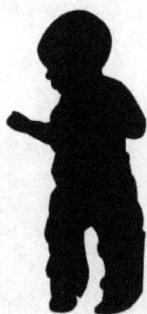

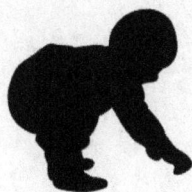

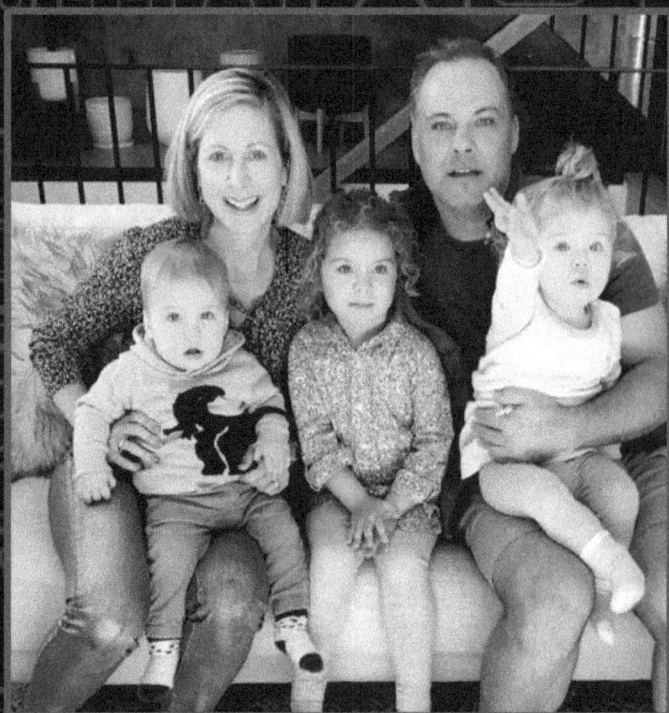
Lisa with her husband and three beautiful children.

I have a few regrets. But living this life and my journey I will never regret. It has been wonderful, amazing and given me the greatest joy. On the other hand, it has been long (so long), devastating, at times lonely and unforgiving. This is my story and I love it!

I am so super proud of what my husband and I have achieved and accomplished. If it wasn't for him, I would not have got through some days and persevered. We were not alone in this journey although we did start the journey that way and that was our choice. Our tribe has always been behind us and given us the strength and courage. Our family and friends have felt our heartache and witnessed the joys and the devastation. When we started out wanting to have a family, we would never have guessed it would have taken so many years, numerous doctor appointments and an overseas expedition to see our dreams come true.

Our story starts like so many others I have spoken to. We met (way too long ago), dated and got married in 2011. We both always wanted kids and had spoken about it before marriage, it was just how many. We started to try for a family and nothing much seemed to happen. I had always had irregular periods and so went and got a checkup at the GP and decided to get a referral at the same time to a fertility specialist. When I finally got into see the fertility specialist, he didn't examine me and just looked over the numerous blood tests that my GP had done. He prescribed Clomid (a medication used to treat infertility in women who do not ovulate) and suggested we 'just keep trying'. So, I went home and took the Clomid and we continued to try. Six months later I fell pregnant, but it wasn't to be.

At the time, I knew something wasn't right so took myself off to the GP and she wanted to get a scan to see if everything was okay. So off I went to have the scan. I will never forget that day.

My husband and I had both planned to attend the scan together but he was unexpectedly called into an urgent meeting and couldn't come. I waited for the appointment wanting to pee the entire time. When they started the scan, they had difficulty in locating the sac as it was so small. Once the sonographer found it, my heart sank as she went quiet, and I just waited for her to tell me that there was no heartbeat.

I was in complete shock and didn't know what to do. The amazing staff guided me and sat with me. I needed to have a D&C (Dilation and Curettage) so they asked me if I knew any obstetricians. I thought of my sister's obstetrician when the staff called her to come up straight away. For a doctor I had never seen she was amazing and to this day I am forever grateful to her. She managed to arrange surgery that evening (it was Good Friday the next day) and I went home packed a bag and went straight to hospital.

That night was extremely hard for my husband and I; we were spending Easter with my parents. We made the decision that we didn't want to ruin the holidays, so we didn't tell anyone. We weren't ready to share our journey yet. So, we grieved in silence.

This time only made us realise how much we wanted kids and we wouldn't stop.

We went back to the obstetrician and she recommended that we see her long-time friend Dr Warren De Ambrosis. To us Warren is a medical and human marvel. That man knows only how to help and guide you on your journey. He gives it to you straight but that is what we wanted. The hours that my husband and I spent with him over the years (and the other amazing doctors and medical professionals that work with him) were some of the happiest and darkest.

No matter what I always appreciated his advice and guidance.

He was there morning, noon and night and never faltered. We've waited for him in the dark for a 5am emergency appointment so worried we couldn't speak to each other, only for him to show up and make us laugh.

Towards the end of 2013 after a miscarriage and three rounds of IUI (intrauterine insemination), I had my first IVF (In Vitro Fertilisation) pickup. Well, didn't that pack a punch. All went well with the pickup and I went home. However in the early hours of the following morning I went to the bathroom and didn't return. My husband found me on the floor and called the ambulance. I had an internal bleed and extremely low blood pressure and needed two blood transfusions.

After this little adventure it was time to tell our parents what we were up to. We are eternally grateful for their support. I recovered and went for the transfer which wasn't successful. The next month we tried another round, first the pickup then the transfer and I fell pregnant. Everything looked fine and I just needed to make it past the six-week mark (so I thought) and all would be OK.

It wasn't to be, even though my HCG (human chorionic gonadotropin) was through the roof. At seven weeks I had some spotting, so we went and saw the doctor. There were two embryo sacs and what looked like a heartbeat but to be sure I needed to rest and come back in a week to check.

The following week my husband and I went to the appointment only to find out there were no heartbeats and I needed another D&C.

The doctor booked me in for the next day.

So, 2013 you can go to hell. Two miscarriages and no kids. As I tried to stay positive all I wanted to do was get back into an IVF cycle and get the ball rolling again. However my body wasn't going to play ball though and I had to wait more than three months before my HCG hormone levels would allow me to start again. We tried everything. My body thought I was pregnant even when I wasn't. I did back-to-back cycles for the rest of the year including scrapings. I even had soy fat pumped into my body to counteract heightened levels of natural killer cells and laparoscopies. My husband and I read so many medical articles and journals, anything we could get our hands on. We told our sisters at Easter that year and our friends what we were going through. They were amazing and completely understanding.

After numerous rounds of IVF throughout the year it was a couple of days before Christmas and after completing another transfer, I felt different, things weren't right.

My sister took me to the doctor and I ended up straight in the hospital with ovarian hyperstimulation. I had blown up like a whale and could hardly breathe there was that much pressure on my lungs. They had to pump protein into me to allow the liquid to drain.

I was in hospital for two weeks over Christmas and New Year's. As horrible as this sounds (and was) on Christmas morning this plight became almost trivial as my husband and I found out I was pregnant, obviously amazing and scary all at the same time. We needed to get past eight weeks. And so, the longest wait in the world began. I also had to rest for the next three months. I took sick leave from work and then arranged to work from home. In August that year it all became worth it, we were blessed with our incredible daughter, Chloe.

We always wanted more than one child and still had frozen embryos so we did not wait too long and started the journey again when I headed back to work the following year. We tried IVF again and after another year-and-a-half and a miscarriage I was told that my body just wasn't going to play ball. I wasn't going to carry another child.

We looked into alternatives and settled on surrogacy. This journey started by needing to arrange for some of our frozen embryos to be shipped overseas. I was grateful that I know my way around documents and was able to arrange for our embryos to be shipped within three weeks. Our surrogacy journey led us down a path where we met an amazing lady on the other side of the world who we are forever grateful and indebted to.

In the middle of that year she went for her first transfer which was successful and she fell pregnant. As a family we travelled to Ukraine in early 2019 a few weeks before our surrogate's due date. We met with our surrogate and settled into our apartment and found our way around Kiev. A week or so later we went to the hospital for the delivery of our baby. Isabella was born and our world changed forever. Chloe became a big sister and Isabella the adorable baby sister.

I tried to breastfeed Isabella, but it wasn't successful due to years of taking medication, so I stopped. Imagine my surprise when I got to bed one night in Kiev and felt something that I was pretty sure I was told I should never feel again. You guessed it! Somehow I was pregnant and the fear set in again. I was on the other side of the world with a three-week-old, our amazing three-year-old and my in-laws who had selflessly come to help us out.

My husband was outside celebrating and drinking shots with them and I couldn't tell him for another two hours. I waited and couldn't go to sleep and told him when he came in. I have never seen anyone jump so high in my life, completely in shock. We made up an excuse to go to the shops the next morning and I got a home pregnancy test. It was positive and then we told my husband's parents. They were overjoyed but at the same time given all my issues and being a geriatric pregnancy there was also fear. We arranged through contacts for me to have an ultrasound and I went the next day. All the results came back fine and so that was a relief.

It was however the shortest pregnancy that we had knowledge of as I was 23 weeks pregnant when we found out.

When we returned to Australia with two kids, I was 25 weeks pregnant. All went well with the pregnancy (even though we only knew about number three for 14 weeks) and our amazing baby boy was born in July 2019.

But Haydn also wanted to have his own dramatic story. Born with breathing difficulties he was taken to the intensive care unit. He was born with underdeveloped lungs which meant he would stay in hospital for a few extra weeks. One of the hardest days yet was walking out of the hospital without a baby to take home and not knowing if he would come home. Within a couple of weeks Haydn made the amazing trip home. We are forever grateful to the incredible team at the Mater Mothers' Neonatal Critical Care Unit.

After more than eight years, 25 IVF procedures, seeing numerous experts, taking numerous drugs (some days more than 20 pills and more than four injections), three miscarriages and three live births (with assistance), we have three amazing kids!

The effect all the medications had on my body was out of this world. I gained 10kgs throughout the entire journey and forget to this day that some people I work with have never known what I [actually] look like! Of course, it is frustrating that my body sometimes faltered but, in the end, it has given us so much.

This journey has not been easy and the emotional toll sometimes suffocating, but I am grateful for the experience and the joy it has brought us. I do not wish this journey on anyone. If there is one lesson that I learnt and will teach my children it is to understand your body, know that not everything can wait and talk about it with others. We need to start the conversation and be proud.

People sometimes ask what got me through the long journey; a couple of quotes that I live by are 'This too shall pass' and 'If at first you don't succeed try and try again'!

Good luck to all, own your journey and know it is your special path. My heart aches for those trying, but know there are many of us that have been there, and we hear your silent prayers.

-Lisa Briese, mother to three beautiful children

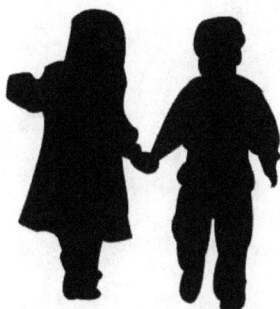

3

Calm after the storm

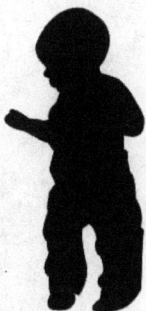

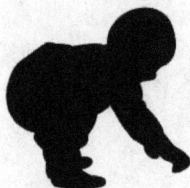

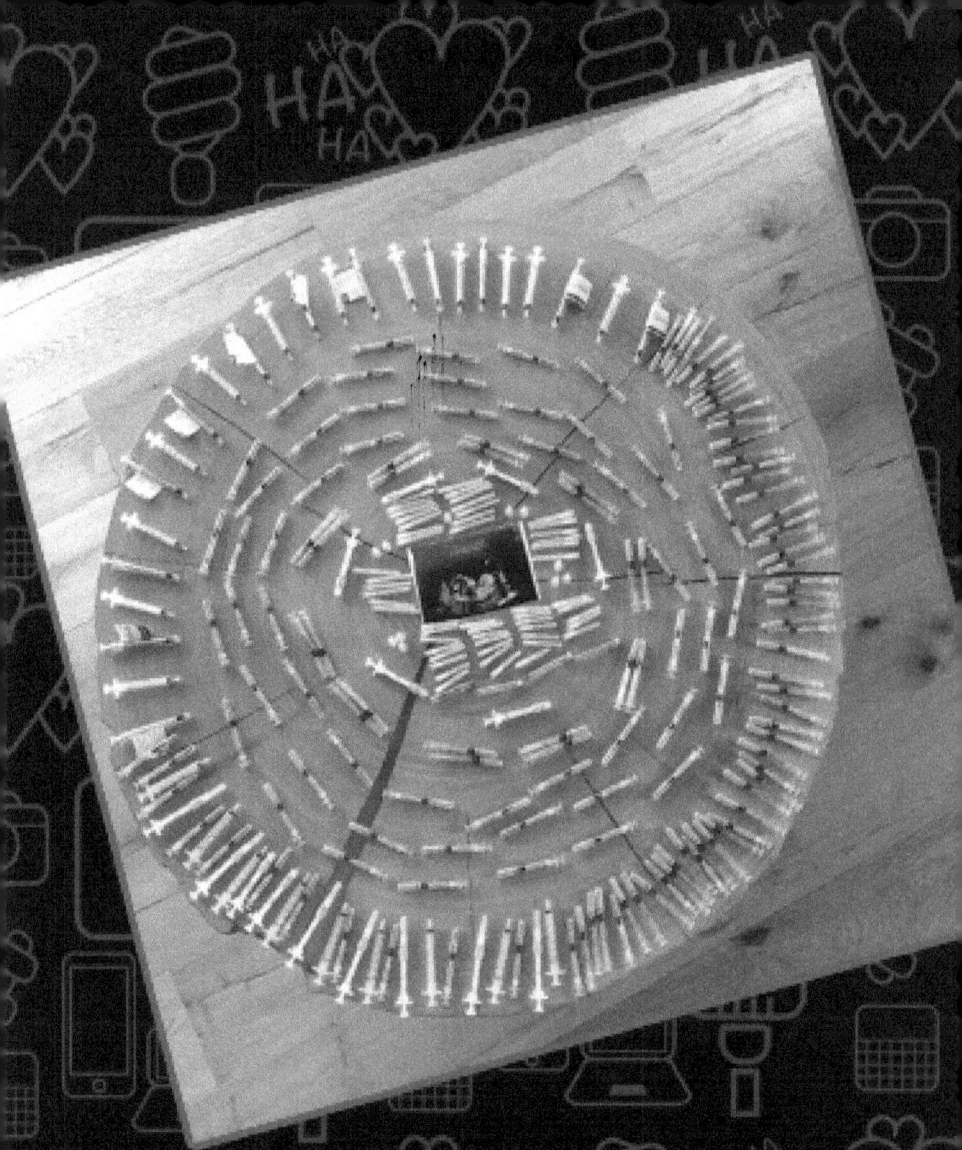

It took numerous hormone injections and lots of medication to receive a much-wanted positive pregnancy result.

In short, two years, two specialists, three full stimulation cycles, several failed FETs (Frozen Embryo Transfers) and a bunch of embryos that did not even get the chance to be transferred. We spent a whole heap of money and rode the emotional rollercoaster we are probably all familiar with to fall pregnant.

Despite what we had to go through, I believe infertility made me become a better mother. I have a great deal of patience and gratitude which I am sure I'd not have had as much of if I conceived quickly and easily.

When I became a mother nearly three years ago (2017), I felt like I was exactly where I needed to be. Some people dream of being pilots, fashion designers, and Olympians but I knew I was put on this earth to be a mum.

The first year of my daughter's life, I was in a blissful little baby bubble, despite sleep deprivation, breastfeeding difficulties, changes in my body and all the other stuff that comes with pregnancy and babies. I loved being a mum.

As our daughter approached a year old, my husband and I discussed a sibling, assuming it would probably take a while again. We made the appointment, made the plan. We had a failed FET and another stim cycle which was cancelled the day before retrieval due to under stimulating. And six months later we were still no closer. Next minute it was the Christmas quiet period, during which no cycles took place.

A new year rolled in, with fresh hope. As one of the first patients back in the door for 2019, I was excited to get going again. I picked up the drugs, and began the stims again. Five days into that cycle, the unimaginable happened. At just over a year-and-half-old, our beautiful IVF miracle girl was diagnosed with cancer.

Without hesitating we cancelled the cycle and informed our wonderful fertility specialist what had happened and focused on getting our daughter better.

Eight months of surgery, chemotherapy, medications, emergency room visits and hospital stays went by slowly. Not much could have made the situation more difficult except for maybe being pregnant and having to be exceptionally cautious with my exposure to oncology medication, or having to care for a new baby as well. So it made me realise in a way that we were lucky nothing had worked so far.

I don't believe that things happen for a reason, but sometimes you can look back and be somehow grateful about it. Hindsight is an interesting thing. I used the forced break from IVF to get myself healthy. I joined a new gym, I put great food into my body 90 per cent of the time, I checked in regularly with my psychologist and obviously, took care of my daughter.

As our daughter was immunocompromised we spent a lot of time at home, and it was nice to have that one-on-one time with her. Her end of treatment scans finally arrived and even more eagerly awaited and hoped for were positive results. Remission!

The final step was a minor surgery and then she would just need regular check-ups for the next five years but her future looked bright. So, we decided to get the IVF ball rolling again, as we had a cruel reminder of how short life can be.

Our fertility specialist convinced us to use our remaining poorly graded embryos in a somewhat impulsive natural FET, which of course did not work.

I felt oddly comforted by the fact that I knew the outcome of those poorly graded embryos that were not even expected to survive the thaw. That in itself gave me hope. I went straight into a new stim cycle (technically the sixth, depending on how you're counting) and a few days before the pregnancy test I came down with a horrendous virus, causing me to cough so much I broke a rib.

How could any embryo possibly survive whatever virus had taken hold of my body? I was so sick and on so many different medications for hormones, supplements as well as antibiotics and painkillers. But to my absolute disbelief, it worked. I was actually pregnant. To this day, I still can't believe how sick I was, and that embryo had stuck.

Morning sickness took hold hard and fast. My daughter was still immunocompromised post-chemo, it worked quite well that we were still basically restricted to the house, with only healthy visitors welcome inside.

It was a difficult pregnancy, the morning sickness (read: all day and night sickness) lasted until the day I gave birth.

My broken rib took ages to heal due to the constant straining from vomiting and the side effects of low iron requiring an infusion to add to the list.

I also had horrendous reflux, constipation, aches all over my body all the time, but I was so glad to be pregnant and so delighted to meet my son or daughter soon.

As our March due date approached, we were getting more excited, however, the news of a new Coronavirus sweeping China was making headlines and as each week came and went the situation seemed to get more dire. "It'll be fine," we kept thinking.

I remember being in the birth suite, with my husband reading the newspaper, which I have kept, and on that date there were 17 pages about Coronavirus. SEVENTEEN! The birth went well and that beautiful little 5AA embryo, the one that stuck there through all that sickness, was a little boy. A son. How completely perfect for us.

But my newborn bubble did not last long this time. While I was lucky that my husband could be with me during labour and in the ward, my daughter was also able to visit, albeit discouraged. Other visitors were also discouraged but allowed as long as they were healthy. But a week later, when I was readmitted due to an unlucky uterine infection, the Australian Government announced massive restrictions to the public. Things were weird. NO visitors were permitted EXCEPT partners and they were asked a series of screening questions upon entry.

Hand sanitisers were zip tied into their holders because they were being stolen. Nurses and midwives were terrified they would be redistributed within the health system. I know in other parts of the world it was even more serious, and my heart goes out to anyone who has to birth alone, or who is facing the prospect of that.

Coming home was tough. We had already spent over a year stuck at home, for fear of what germs could seriously harm our daughter. We had already done the chalk drawings on the footpath, made the play dough and the finger painting. We had done the social isolation thing, but that time we had support.

We had grandparents coming over to fold a pile of washing. We had cousins coming over to play. We had friends dropping in with meals and new books/toys to entertain us. This time we had none of that. Plus a newborn. So many things that I had planned to make this transition easy for all of us, were ripped out from underneath us.

Due to social distancing rules, it also meant mothers groups were cancelled, baby health clinics were cancelled, grandma was NOT allowed to hold the baby, and coffee with a friend was cancelled too.

You need some toilet paper? Too bad, the supermarket had sold out - should have bought some earlier. And don't bother trying online delivery because that was cancelled too.

Newborns were not even permitted at a mother's six-week obstetric check—up, so with a toddler and no support, even mundane but 'essential' activities such as medical appointments became a logistical nightmare.

I have spoken of feeling like I was between a rock and a hard place because at times, that's what it was.

I have talked passionately about how worried I am for the mental health of new parents and pregnant people during this time, as I feel we've been overlooked as we are not sick or elderly. So many avenues of support were taken from us, not to mention levels of anxiety that come with becoming new parents. Throw anxiety that comes with a pandemic on top of that, and it's a recipe for disaster.

After a lot of thought and discussion with a mental health professional, I realised the reason why I was so upset by all this and struggling with it was because I was struck with grief.

I was grieving what could have been, what I was lucky enough to have with my first, and what I won't get again. I feel like the fast flying newborn weeks and the beautiful bubble that comes with it was like a carpet that was ripped out from under my feet.

I felt similarly when I began my IVF journey and learned that I would never have a late period, pee on a stick, and have that magic surprise fairytale moment. I grieved not being able to have the conception most women dream their whole lives of, that so many do get. In some ways going through infertility and IVF taught me how to cope with grief, especially the weird kind where you never really had anything to lose in the first place, but just the idea of something that felt so real.

I am also trying not to find silver linings in this because for me that just forces me to feel better when I am not ready — grief takes time.

I do want to say that I am grateful that I get this time to cuddle my baby boy all to myself. That we get to figure this out as a family and that we have plenty of time to do it. I am grateful he has not had the opportunity to be exposed to other pathogens that aren't Covid-19, but other scary ones that can be very dangerous to newborns.

And most of all, pandemic or no pandemic, I am grateful he is here - my little lockdown baby, my miracle.

If you find yourself grieving during this pandemic whether it be an actual loss, or something less tangible such as time because you now have to wait for fertility treatment to start again, or the idea of what you had planned for your baby to start life did not eventuate, financial loss, or maybe even just the loss of normalcy and routine, my heart goes out to you.

And know this. You are not alone. We are not all in the same boat but we are all in the same storm, and it's a scary storm. Your feelings are valid. It is important to reach out to someone, a friend or professional, if you need help processing it.

Also remember, this too shall pass. Restrictions are now easing rapidly in parts of the country though it may be some time until things are back to "normal", whatever that will be, but it will pass. And boy, we will be a resilient bunch of people on the other side of it.

- **Anonymous**

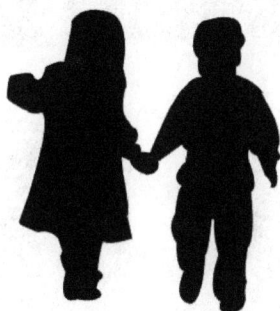

4

Saying goodbye

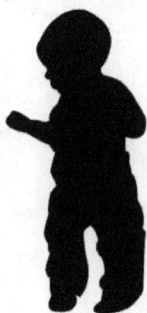

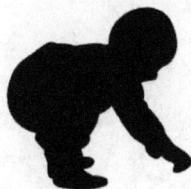

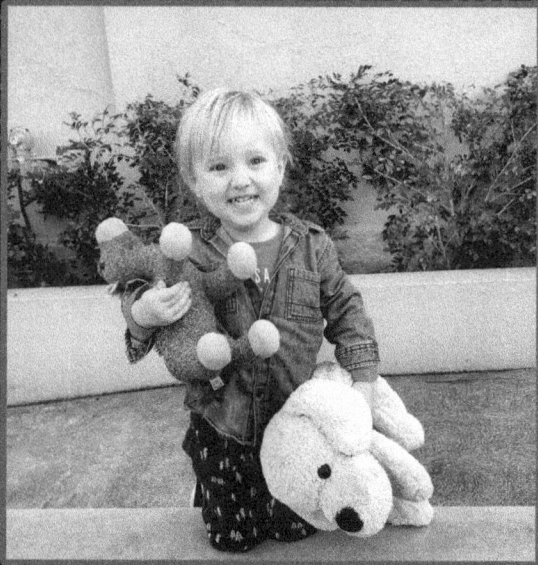
Kingsley is a cheeky and fun- loving little boy.

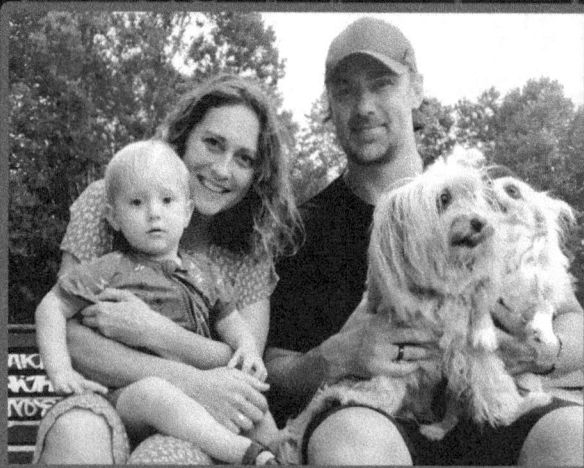
Vanessa and Woody with their son Kingsley and
beloved dogs Charlton and Fox.

Making the decision to terminate our pregnancy, to end the unrealised life of our baby girl, will forever be a source of pain and torment.

After lovingly growing our child for 16 weeks, saying the words "we have chosen to terminate" was the most difficult I have ever spoken. To actually say them aloud and confirm our decision to the genetics counsellors - who had been with us when we first discovered my partner's condition - was almost impossible.

It meant ending the dream of introducing our daughter to her older brother, our outrageously wonderful Kingsley, of caring for her as we had him and making her part of our family. "You didn't have a choice," we have been told by so many people and while deep down I know this to be true, it doesn't lessen the sorrow I carry with me every day.

In 2017, my partner, Woody, and I discovered we were pregnant with our first child. Despite the chronic morning sickness and fatigue, we assumed everything was normal. We were oblivious to the fact Woody was living with a genetic condition that, if passed on, would be a devastating diagnosis for any of his children.

Seven weeks into the pregnancy, Woody and I were in our car about to leave home when his back started to spasm. After 45 minutes of lying on the road doing gentle stretches, I was able to support him back inside the house. The next day I walked him to a doctor a couple of minutes from our place, needless to say, he was in a seriously sorry state.

She noticed things on Woody's body—dark patches and random growths on his skin – and since he had mentioned we were expecting, she wasted no time referring him to a dermatologist. In the past, Woody had these things looked at by doctors but they were never investigated. This particular doctor had insight and an understanding if he had what she suspected, there were genetic implications for our baby.

Blood tests confirmed her suspicions but the result was far from expected. Woody was found to have an extremely rare occurrence of neurofibromatosis 1 (NF1) – put basically, a genetic disorder that causes tumours to form on nerve tissue such as in the brain and spinal cord. This condition was most commonly a result of a genetic mutation however, Woody's presents as a gene deletion in a mosaic pattern, something we were told at the time had only been discovered in eight other people in the world.

We were told because of the rarity, doctors had no idea of the chances of this being passed on but if it was, there would be gene deletions in the baby's entire body. We had to find out if our child was affected but first a specific genetic test had to be developed in a specialist laboratory in Alabama, USA. Weeks past and at 20 weeks, I went in for an amniocentesis – where a needle was inserted into the uterus to extract amniotic fluid containing the baby's DNA.

Our care from doctors and specialists at the Royal Hospital for Women in Randwick, Sydney, was incredible. They sat with us and went through all known possibilities and helped Woody get tests to search his body for tumours. We were told many adults with NF1 would start to go blind as tumours can grow on optic nerves.

They checked for this and to our relief, no tumours were found. They did find a growth in his brain but assured us it was only something to watch, not act on.

At 22 weeks' gestation we drove to the hospital for the results of the amniocentesis. After preparing for the worst we received the best possible news. Our baby was going to be OK. Despite a complicated birth at 41 weeks where, after being induced and a day of labour, our son's shoulders became stuck behind my pubic bones in what is called shoulder dystocia, a healthy and heavy Kingsley was born.

After two years of getting to know our wonderful, cheeky and hilariously delightful son, we fell pregnant again. As everything was great with Kingsley, we expected the same for baby number two. The testing happened quicker this time but the weeks were slow and worrisome as we were unsure what they would reveal.

I went for my initial dating scan alone as I was visiting family in Tasmania and remember seeing the tiny heartbeat and feeling overjoyed but at the same time terrified. Having known Kingsley and realising this child was his little brother or sister created an unexpected array of emotions. We knew if Woody's condition were to be passed on, it would not present in a way NF1 tends to.

Our greatest fears were realised when testing found 21 genes were deleted from our child.

We had undertaken a Chorionic villus sampling (CVS), a test carried out during pregnancy to detect specific abnormalities in an unborn baby. A sample of cells is taken from the placenta and tested for genetic defects.

Without going into too much detail, the child would have had numerous issues.

We wanted our baby so badly. I asked our genetics counsellor what her life would be like. He told us people who he has treated with NF1 are happy to be alive but live difficult lives and because of the severity of her condition, the life our baby faced would be extremely unpleasant, painful and most likely short. Even writing this makes me feel like a horrible person and I am terrified to tell our story to those not in our immediate circle. It was a choice we had to make for not only our baby girl but for Kingsley.

I have only told my partner this but I gave her the name, Aphra, which means from the earth.

One year has passed since she was cremated and talking about it still causes me to internally freeze. I had complications following the procedure where a scan located retained products of conception (RPOC) with a blood source present in my uterus. I had been experiencing heavy periods with lots of clotting and was often unwell with symptoms of nausea, tiredness and swelling in my uterus and arms and legs. Eight months after the medical termination, I was back in hospital to have my uterus assessed. After expecting scarring and lesions from the RPOC, my uterus was found to be in a good condition and whatever was in there had made its way out.

We have now started down the IVF route and are in the process of having a specific genetic test created to have embryos assessed before implantation. Aphra's results will help make that possible.

The pre-implantation genetic testing and IVF path is expensive and I am to understand wreaks havoc with hormones but for us, it is the best option. If to happen naturally, we have been told any future pregnancy has a 50 per cent chance of genetic deletions occurring. It is a game of Russian roulette we wish not to play ever again.

-Vanessa Croll

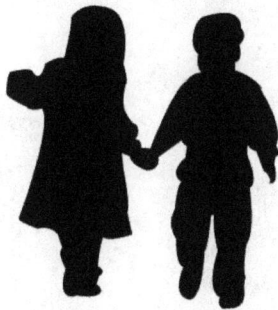

5

Navigating life beyond NICU

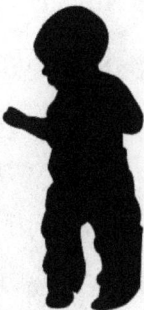

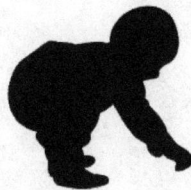

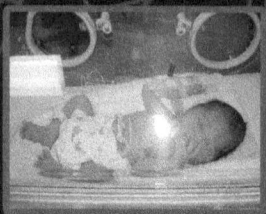
Elijah Cruz in hospital.

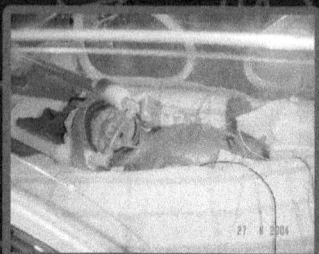
Dillon Cruz's first day in hospital.

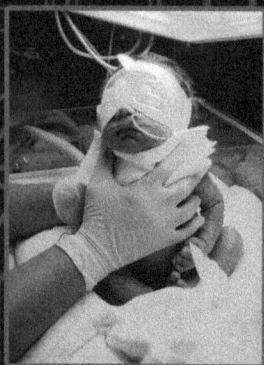
Jasper Cruz in hospital.

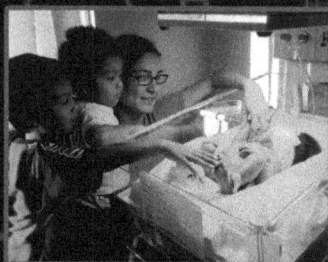
Melinda Cruz with her two older sons meeting Jasper.

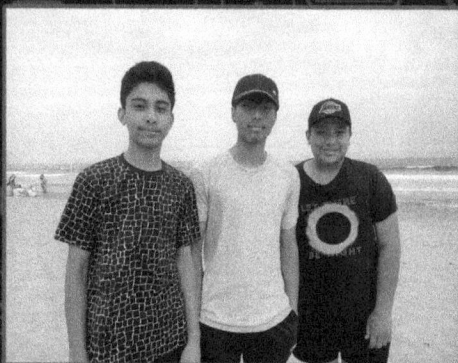
The Cruz boys several years on.

At 18, I was diagnosed with a bicornuate uterus and endometriosis and told that I would find it hard to either fall pregnant, stay pregnant or I would have my babies early.

At 24, I was so excited to be pregnant with my first son. It happened very quickly and after a small bleed at six weeks which resolved itself, my pregnancy ran smoothly. That is until 29 weeks when I started having contractions. I was hospitalised and put on bedrest. Three weeks later my waters broke, not completely, but I was leaking amniotic fluid. I managed to hold on to him for another two weeks and delivered him at 34 weeks. He was immediately taken to the Neonatal Intensive Care Unit (NICU).

Just over a year later, I was pregnant again. This time my plan was to get to 29 weeks and then go onto bedrest. Unfortunately, that did not happen and at 27 weeks I went into labour and it could not be stopped. I delivered another beautiful little boy. He was resuscitated and taken to the NICU.

When pregnant with my third son, my doctor decided he would put in a cervical stitch in the hope it would help me hold him a little longer. The procedure was performed when I was 12 weeks pregnant and although I needed to be on bedrest from 23 weeks, the stitch worked and I carried him to almost 37 weeks. Due to developing jaundice, he was also admitted into the NICU for a short stay.

In total, my boys spent nearly 13 weeks in NICU. It was probably the most scared I have ever been in my life and the experience changed me forever. It didn't get easier when we were home especially with my 27 weeker as we knew that we may have challenges with his development.

It was during this time and whilst trying to navigate our life beyond the NICU that I initiated the idea of the Miracle Babies Foundation. Having contact with other families who had been there as well as access to long term support and services had a huge impact on my sons' outcomes, along with the way I was able to cope with their traumatic early arrivals.

Now running for 15 years, the Foundation is here to support families of premature and sick babies and my boys are amazing, healthy teenagers. Every year in Australia around 48,000 newborn babies require the help of a Neonatal Intensive Care Unit or Special Care Nursery. About 27,000 of these babies are born premature and up to 1000 babies lose their fight for life.

For families, the experience of having a baby come into the world not as expected or planned is life changing. Without support, this overwhelming and traumatic experience can have lifelong effects on the emotional wellbeing of these miracle families. It affects the entire family unit.

Australia is home to 23 state-of-the-art intensive care units designed to meet the unique and critical needs of our earliest and sickest babies. Working with health professionals on the joint agenda of better outcomes for families, Miracle Babies provides informative education and insight on a family's experience and funding for equipment, resources and research.

I would never have chosen the way my babies came into the world and the way they had to fight for life, but when I look back at the options I was given by my doctors and the follow on effect of the creation of Miracle Babies Foundation helping so many other families like mine,

I can definitely see that in my heartache was the greatest blessing.

**- Melinda Cruz, Miracle Babies Foundation founder,
Visit www.miraclebabies.org.au**

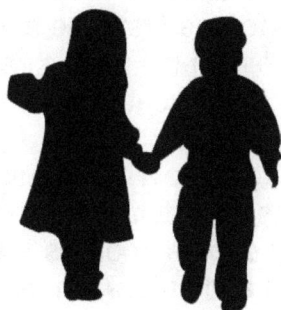

6

Triple the fun

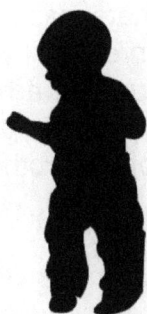

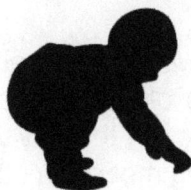

I was born at 24 weeks weighing just 900g. I was one of triplets born in August 1990. My brothers and I were fighters from the start. I stayed in hospital for three months before going home for the first time and my mother and father couldn't nurse me until I was three months old because my skin was too delicate.

I kept fighting and grew into a healthy adult. I'm very sensitive to the cold as an adult and I think this is due to being in a humidity crib as soon as I was born, always wanting to be warm and safe. I am thankful for my birth story because it makes me the strong woman I am today.

However there is a twist to my story.

When my brothers and I were born, mum and dad had to adopt out the sickest of the three of us, because he needed 24-hour care. My brother who was adopted out was in hospital for 18 months before going home for the first time. Growing up I did not know this part of my story, I thought I was a twin.

When I was 16, mum shared with me that I was actually a triplet and that I in fact had another brother. I was so grateful to find out that he had grown up into a healthy and beautiful individual. I felt so happy that the doctors and nurses had taken such good care of my brother and he had survived too.

My two brothers and I were reunited when we were 17 years old. It was absolutely amazing to suddenly be a triplet. On the day we first met, my brothers without ever having met each other, wore the same style of clothes —

black jeans, a white collared shirt and a suit jacket. They even ordered the same thing at lunch.

Within a week of meeting one another, my brothers and I were playing music and singing with perfect natural harmonies. It was as if we had been practising music together forever. Our friends and family were blown away by the instant connection that we all had as triplets.

Before meeting one another, the brother who I grew up with could not play guitar or sing, whereas I had always been musically inclined. It was absolutely mind blowing and also like a miracle that after reuniting, my brother could suddenly play the guitar without any formal training, and less than one week of practice.

To this day, we are healthy young adults, against all odds.

-The author of this story is now aged 30 and wishes to remain anonymous.

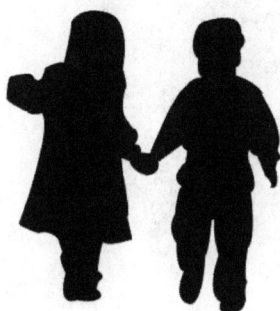

7

Living an alternate reality

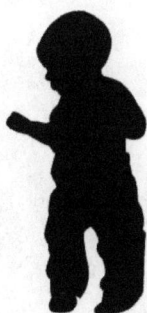

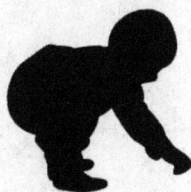

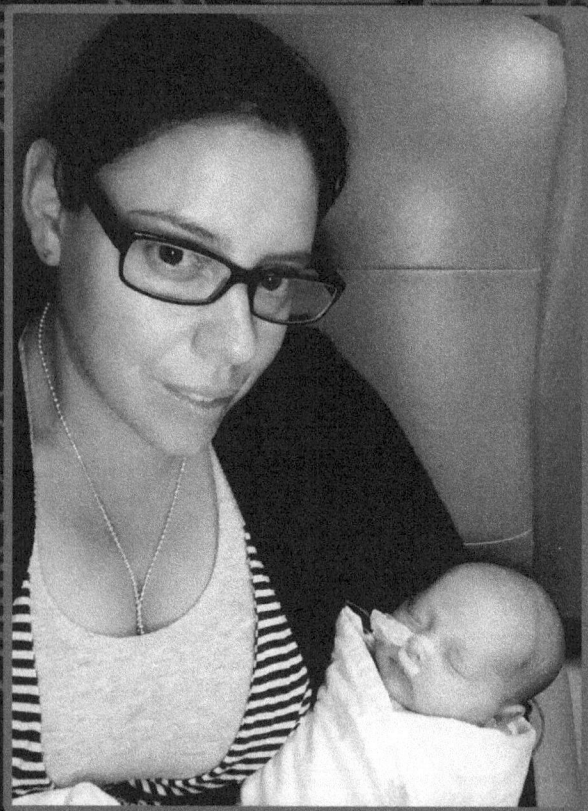
Sarah with her daughter Lily.

Lily was brought onto this earth to challenge my plans; and as a person who demands control and order, this has been and will continue to be a learning curve. After many years of trying unsuccessfully to conceive, I had lost hope that I would experience motherhood. Subsequently, making the conscious choice to focus on my career, rather than my failed attempts at entering parenthood, I accepted a senior role at a new company and relocated interstate. Two months later, I discovered I was pregnant.

Lily Mihiarangi Whelan made her entrance into this world —six weeks early and ready to challenge the world. The birth was undoubtedly not to plan, but Lily and I were happy and healthy.

Notwithstanding, Lily spent four weeks in the special care nursery. During that time, I was living an alternate reality, arriving at the hospital each morning, inhabiting a small room, where I watched protectively over Lily in her little incubator, and later a tiny bassinet. Babies came and went. Excited parents left with their new babies while I sat quietly in the corner. I spent days reading, more often than not attached to an electric breast pump, until late at night when the nurses would encourage me to leave for the day. As a mother of a premature baby, I felt powerless.

There was never a thought that Lily would not be breast-fed. But life had other plans, my milk had not come in, and Lily was supplied with formula. Thus, my battle with my milk supply began.

They say that once you have had a baby, all your inhibitions float out the window. I think they are still there, but you put them aside for your new priorities.

So, if I needed to (awkwardly) sit with a boob exposed so that one of the nurses could squeeze a few drops for Lily – sign me up. A few drops led to a few more. I was then introduced to an electric breast pump. I was diligent in expressing both sides, every two hours for twenty minutes. But for all the effort, I felt I was not providing enough.

"Strength and growth come only through continuous effort and struggle" - Napoleon Hill.

The nurses provided insights into foods and natural remedies that could help boost my milk production. I was introduced to fenugreek, brewers yeast, oats and apricots. One of the special care nurses recommended 'boobie biscuits'. My mum found a recipe online, and these little morsels were my go-to pre-pump snack. After another week of relentless expressing and boobie biscuits, the doctors prescribed me Motilium. Also referred to as Domperidone, the medication increases the level of the hormone prolactin which is involved in breast milk production. Expressing or breastfeeding frequently, while taking domperidone, will help increase breast milk supply.

Finally, I was able to start feeding Lily solely on breast milk (through her nasal tube). Not quite to plan, but getting closer. Over the next few weeks, I was able to keep up with Lily's needs; and was able to start stockpiling a small number of reserves. No matter how much milk I produced, I was convinced that I could not make enough.

In true Sarah-style, I started over-analysing the situation. I tracked how much milk I was able to provide, how much stored, how much milk Lily currently needed, how much she would need next week. I set myself goals on how much I wanted to produce. But milk supply is not achieved by setting goals, motherhood is not about setting KPIs.

The matter was compounded by the fact that Lily was a little baby. Although healthy and happy and meeting her development milestones, Lily was in the lowest percentile on the growth and weight charts. I attributed this slow growth to my inability to provide enough milk; a massive cloud of uncertainty encumbered me.

I continued to bottle feed Lily with expressed breast milk; I was so nervous that if I switched to breastfeeding, I would not be able to satiate Lily's needs. I have learned that self-doubt is a side-effect of parenthood. I expressed continually. The low thrum of the little motor was my background music. I expressed in mother's rooms, department store change rooms and the back of the car. I felt like this small yellow device was an extension of me.

When Lily was four months old, I tried breastfeeding – actual breastfeeding. Success! Lily took to the boob like a fish to water. I loved it. Finally, I was experiencing the motherhood I had envisioned.

But Lily continued to sit at the lowest percentage of the growth chart. I became paranoid that maybe it wasn't just my supply, perhaps it was the quality of my milk. I spent eight months over analysing and criticising myself about my inability to be the type of mother I had wanted.

The problem was, nobody had indicated to me how much milk was sufficient. When Lily was nine months old, I made the decision to switch to formula. I was defeated, I could not perform to the level that I required of myself.

"Though she be but little, she be fierce" – Shakespeare

Coincidentally, Lily did not put on weight nor grow at a faster rate with formula. She still sits on the lower percentile of the growth chart. I was so preoccupied with my own insecurities that I lost perspective. Nonetheless, we made it through the first year. Lily, a fearless ball of energy, has taught me to be kinder to myself. I now am happy to let myself get lost in the moment and enjoy my beautiful family.

- Sarah Whelan

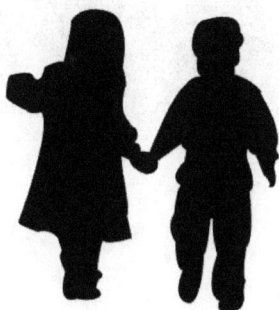

8

Mother's milk - a life saviour

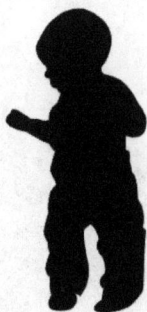

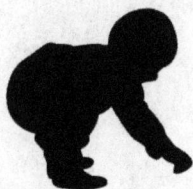

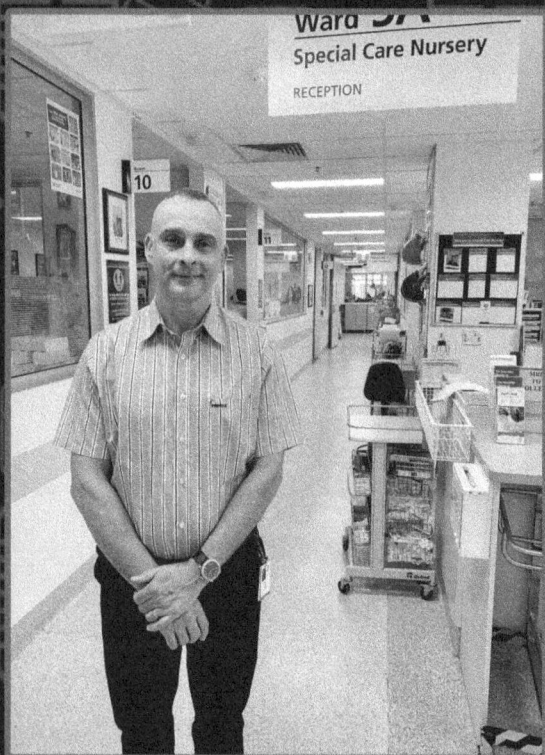

Dr Pieter Koorts, director of the Queensland Milk Bank at The Royal Brisbane and Women's Hospital (RBWH), and director of Neonatology

Dr Pieter Koorts is the director of the Queensland Milk Bank (QMB) at The Royal Brisbane and Women's Hospital (RBWH), and director of Neonatology.

It is universally accepted that breast milk is the optimum exclusive source of nutrition for infants. This holds even more true for preterm infants where exclusive human milk feeds protect preterm infants from a range of life-threatening conditions, including a devastating gut condition called necrotizing enterocolitis, as well as hospital acquired infection.

In fact, a preterm baby fed cows milk formula instead of their mother's own milk or donor milk has double the risk of developing necrotizing enterocolitis. An all-human milk diet can also lead to improved neurodevelopmental outcomes and improved visual development in preterm babies.

Despite best efforts, a mother's own milk is not always available for a variety of reasons. In studies, up to a third of mothers were unable to sustain their lactation to meet their premature infants' needs during the first couple of weeks. The reasons may vary from geographical isolation, especially in such a large country like Australia, to maternal illness and stress of having a preterm baby admitted to a neonatal intensive care unit. Avoiding the use of formula in preterm babies by using Pasteurised Donor Human Milk (PDHM) is a very cost-effective strategy that has received increased attention during the last decade in Australia.

Pasteurised donor milk is obtained from a human milk bank, an organisation established for the purpose of enrolling and collecting excess breastmilk from non-remunerated donors. It is then processed, tested, stored and distributed as a safe and suitable human milk to recipients that are not the donor's own infants, to meet their specific needs for optimal health. It does not include informal milk sharing that occurs in the community. Wet nursing has occurred throughout the ages well into the 20th century, to be replaced by informal milk banks located in hospitals. These were mostly closed in the 1980s with the advent of HIV and the recognition that raw human milk can transmit infectious diseases.

It took until the 2000s for human milk banking to be reignited in Australia, with the first milk bank opening in Perth, utilising the traditional method of Holden pasteurisation (heating milk to 62.5C for 30 minutes) to safeguard the milk from a microbiological point of view. Since then a small number of milk banks have opened across Australia, including the RBWH Milk Bank, which opened in November 2012, with milk donated from a bereaved donor. Without those precious 40 litres, the milk bank may never have opened.

Compared with the USA and Europe, there is still an inequity of access to donor milk across Australia. RBWH eventually morphed into the Queensland Milk Bank as they started supplying more hospitals around the state and across the country as far as Tasmania.

The QMB reached 1000 donors in 2020 and has pasteurised and distributed more than 8000 litres since opening. One litre can meet the needs of 50 babies as many preterm babies only start on 1ml every three hours, which means a litre of liquid gold as it is often called, can go a long way.

Due to the complex and necessary safety steps that we must go through to ensure that the milk is as safe as it can be, it is a very scarce and expensive resource. This means that PDHM is only used in babies where there is a proven (by rigorous studies) benefit for its use.

The most robust evidence for the use of PDHM is in preterm babies (less than 34 weeks or less than 1,500) as a substitute for cows milk formula where mother's own milk is not available. It is not a replacement for a mother's own milk and should only be part of a package of support for lactation, or as a crutch to support mother's own milk feeding.

There is very little evidence that PDHM confers any benefit to term babies over the use of formula and the prohibitive cost means that it should be reserved for preterm babies at this stage.

There is some research ongoing to find out whether there are other groups of infants who may benefit from PDHM, like larger babies who are infants of diabetic mothers and the late preterm babies (24-37 weeks' gestation).

Milk banks have well thought out processes in order to ensure absolute safety of the milk that we then feed to small, vulnerable babies, some of which may weight a mere 500 grams. Donors are asked to complete a life-style and risk assessment questionnaire, very similar to when you donate blood. Every donor will have bloods done, testing for transmittable diseases like HIV, hepatitis and syphilis. A detailed medication history is important, as some medications can get excreted into the breast milk, which may affect small babies (not necessarily a mother's own term baby). Once the donor is approved and a substantial donation is made, the milk is checked for any bacteria growing in the milk. It is then pasteurised and checked again for bacteria. Any milk growing a large number of bacteria is discarded. Only when all the above are signed off is the milk made available for use. It can be stored frozen for three months after processing.

The QMB currently supplies milk to 14 intensive care and special care nurseries across Queensland and Tasmania. The parents of the babies receiving the milk do not have to pay for the milk, it is covered by the hospitals. The hospitals will have very strict criteria for the use of PDHM as it is so expensive a resource. It costs around $300 per litre for the whole process. The cost savings for preterm babies and the reduction in complications make that investment very worthwhile though. We are always looking for ways to improve the outcomes for babies and for ways to bring liquid gold to more babies across Australia.

Find out more via the Queensland Milk Bank's Facebook page.

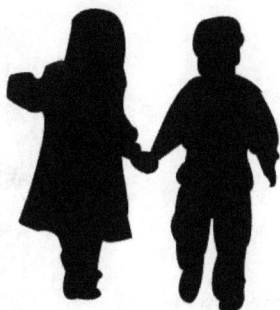

9

Helping the smallest of fighters

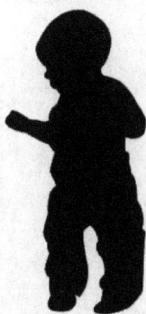

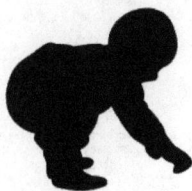

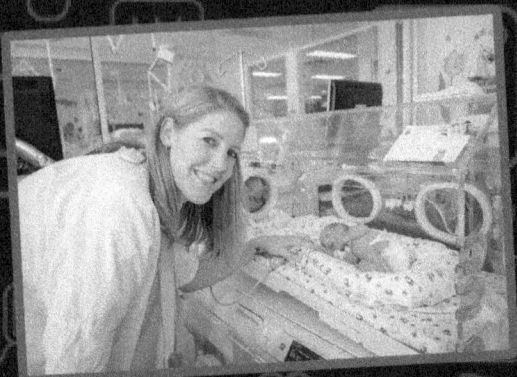

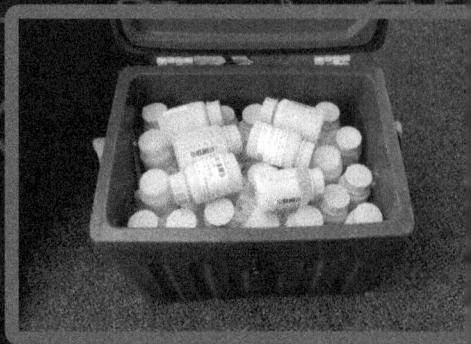

Queensland
MILKBANK

With Special Thanks

Nicola Rigby

You have kindly donated more than 50.8 litres of Breastmilk and have
helped babies throughout Queensland, New South Wales
and Tasmania.

_____   _____
Milk Bank Director   Milk Bank Manager

'Saving the lives of our very finiest Queenslanders'

Our baby Elsie was born on February 28, 2017 at 30+1 weeks' gestation. Our stay in the NICU/SCN (Neonatal Intensive Care Unit/Special Care Nursery) was relatively uneventful and we were home at 36+3 weeks' gestation.

Elsie was born early as I had a shortened cervix. She weighed 1526g at birth. I was away from home, Charleville, for a total of two months. I expressed three to four hourly around the clock until Elsie was exclusively breastfed from 36 weeks, then I would express morning and night.

I donated roughly half my supply while Elsie was in hospital and only took a limited supply home with us. I donated my frozen breast milk a number of times when we travelled to Brisbane for her check-ups. I would fly to Brisbane and my breastmilk was checked in as premium hand luggage to help keep it from defrosting.

I chose to donate to give something back to the hospital that helped our baby. I felt like it was the least I could do considering all they'd done for Elsie. Having previously worked at the RBWH (Royal Brisbane and Women's Hospital) as a midwife years ago, I felt a real connection to the hospital. I felt great pride in donating my breastmilk knowing it was helping the smallest of fighters.

-Nicola Rigby, human milk donor for the Queensland Milk Bank

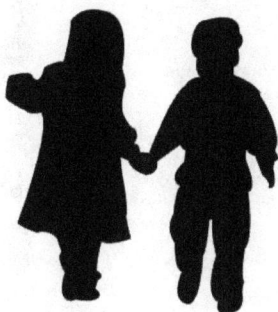

10

Our NICU rollercoaster

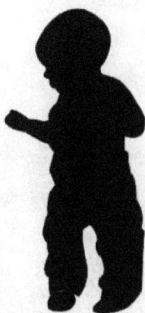

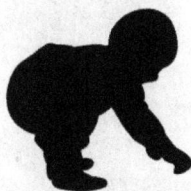

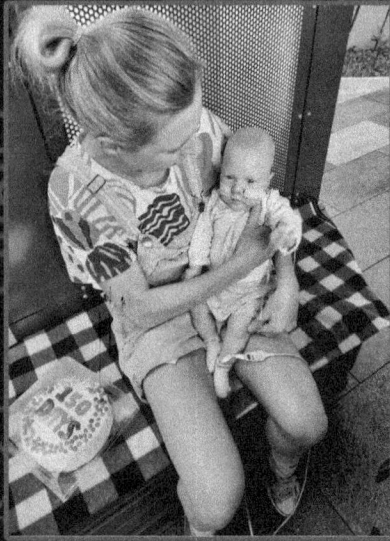
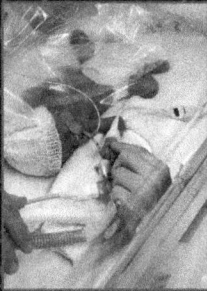
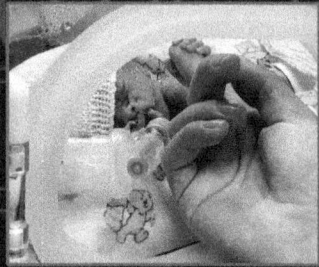

Summer was born at 729g and has shown not only her parents but her doctors and nurses her fighting spirit despite more than 150 days in hospital

Dear beautiful and ever amazing Summer, (also known as Sum-Sum).

This is not the way we had things planned. We should have been hanging out at the beach, enjoying nature and playing with your puppy. I see you staring out your window at the big blue sky and know you should be getting out amongst it and exploring the world. Nevertheless, I would hardly believe how far you've come except I've sat next to your incubator, open cot and now big girl cot for more than 150 days and witnessed your amazing strength.

I hope this letter can somewhat demonstrate your resilience and that if you're ever afraid or doubting your ability, you can reflect on all that you achieved before your first step.

In retrospect, being born and taking a breath was a huge achievement. In those couple of days when we understood not all was right, doctors would comment how strong your heart was, and despite being in a hostile environment, you remained very settled. Still, the official term used to describe you was "scrawny".

We were given the information (on issues) of having a baby born at 27 weeks' gestation, however, we took more notice of the 28 week one that had improved odds.

With something also identified as "not being right with your bowel", the medical staff prepared for the likelihood of you having cystic fibrosis (two genetic tests and a sweat test later, that was not the case).

So even before coming into the world, we were already facing some significant battles together.

I desperately wanted to keep you in, but on the morning of May 11, 2020 my body was not cooperating and the obstetrician, looking out for both of us, decided it was time.

It was all so surreal, business-like, waiting our turn to be wheeled into the operating theatre knowing we were only minutes away from meeting you. Daddy got to meet you minutes later but it was hours for me.

I missed you in my tummy from the moment you left. Reassuringly you squawked on the way out and gave it your very best on the 'snorkel' before needing a breathing tube in. Over the next few days I would only see you for snippets of the day, daddy a little more. The nurses called you feisty itsy-bitsy and that indeed has rung true every day thereafter.

When you were three days old we found out your bowel was misbehaving and so you would need to move hospitals. Less than an hour later you were packed into your rocket ship and on your way. We were in shock, I was in shock as at 7pm that night I was still at RBWH (Royal Brisbane and Women's Hospital) and you were across town, about to go into surgery.

All on your own. I am so sorry. You were so very brave. Again the anaesthetist commented on how feisty you were and you came through surgery amazingly well. Knowing now the nurses who sent you off and helped you recover, you were in very good hands.

After spending much time in NICU, I've seen many bubs arrive without their mummas and it broke my heart every time. Knowing how I felt and sometimes seeing mummas not being able to be with their unwell baby for many days was cruel and torturous.

While recovery from surgery went well, your little lungs were just not quite ready for the outside world and after having the breathing tube out for several days, fatigue set in and thus the tube was needed again. Soon after, the first sepsis came about and the bug also headed into your lungs. This was just after we'd celebrated you reaching 1kg. We were so excited and had cake as NICU tradition goes.

There were some tough days on the ventilator and turns out you were tougher... or again feisty, and you kept fighting the ventilator. Because you have grown bigger, you got another trial off it but again your little lungs were too little and stiff, so the tube went back in. A course of steroids combined with high dose caffeine, eventually helped you kick the ventilator. Once the steroids wore off, things got tough again but late one Friday night your fighting spirit and one of many blood transfusions helped bolster you up enough to keep the doctors at bay. After weeks on the snorkel, you breezed onto high flow (a form of non-invasive respirator support) and it looked like we were finally moving forward. But then your tummy played tricks again and devastatingly rather, than going for the planned ileostomy reversal (an ileostomy is used to move waste out of the body, the surgery is done when the colon or rectum does not work properly), we walked you back to the operating theatre for emergency surgery just in time, as your heart and lungs were starting to feel the effects.

We hoped your bowel could be reconnected, but it was not to be so a new stoma was formed. Your lungs took a massive hit, and for a couple of days there I prayed with you, held your hand and held my tears (most of) for when not in the room. I knew how tough you were, but watching the neonatologist sitting with you for much of the day, everyone's faces in NICU and the constant beeping of the irritating monitors, started to eat at my strength. Not yours however. All the fluid started to shift and your lungs re-inflated. Five days later you got the breathing tube out —still very tough going but twice daily physio and very patient doctors meant it stayed out.

Eventually you returned to being the "boring baby" — a very good thing in NICU.

The NICU roller coaster is a beast, and after arriving for another day, we checked your temperature and it was 39.4C. Another sepsis, not a nice bug (are any?), and in retrospect the doctor commented that you evaded getting really sick. You showed your strength by actually weaning oxygen and improving your feeding. I also think you had someone looking out for you. Between these larger events, you've endured many smaller ones including lumbar punctures, contrast studies, PICC (peripherally inserted central catheter) insertions, so many cannulations, blood and plasma transfusions, head ultrasound, ECHOs — all without fuss, just with your "ninja hands" at the ready.

Sharing your journey with you has been the hardest but most amazing thing I've been through. It's important to note that the intensity of the NICU rollercoaster needs to also take into account the many babies and families the ride is shared with.

Intentional and not, for even if you block your ears and look away, it's impossible to ignore what is going on around you. When your neighbour has the privacy screens put up and multitudes of visitors in a no visitor COVID policy, it's easy to recognise it's not a good outcome. With families that you choose to share your story, it is an amazing source of comfort and support.

But be warned, share the joy of small and big wins and be prepared to feel the angst and pain when things aren't going so well.

To the extent of watching the heartbreaking funeral (online) of your (Summer's) little mate — we'll never forget him or his most beautiful strong parents.

Your nurses (aunties) took the greatest of care of you. And us. They too cheered you on, held your hand. It's always the smaller things —special name tag, homemade sheets, sneaky chocolates, pep talks, hugs (shh) and on more than one occasion 'Summer just didn't seem herself so I...'. They knew you, they also rode your journey with you, they loved you too. Several neonatologists said "your Summer has had a tough trot even by NICU standards". I wish that weren't true, but it is undeniable. Really then, it points to your toughness, resilience and spirit and amplified with all the prayers, love and positive energy that friends and family have sent.

Our journey is not over, and I'm praying the rollercoaster is slightly less bumpy going forward. Either way, I have true belief that you'll not just be okay, you are and will be AMAZING.

- **Love you to the moon and back, mumma xxx, Stella Foley**

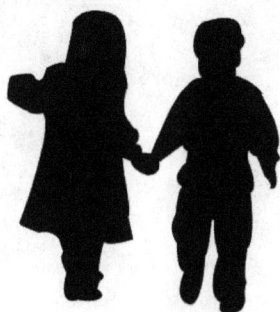

11

Experiencing NICU

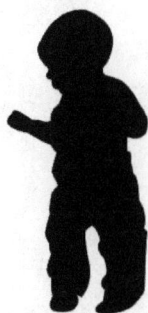

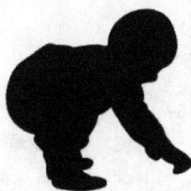

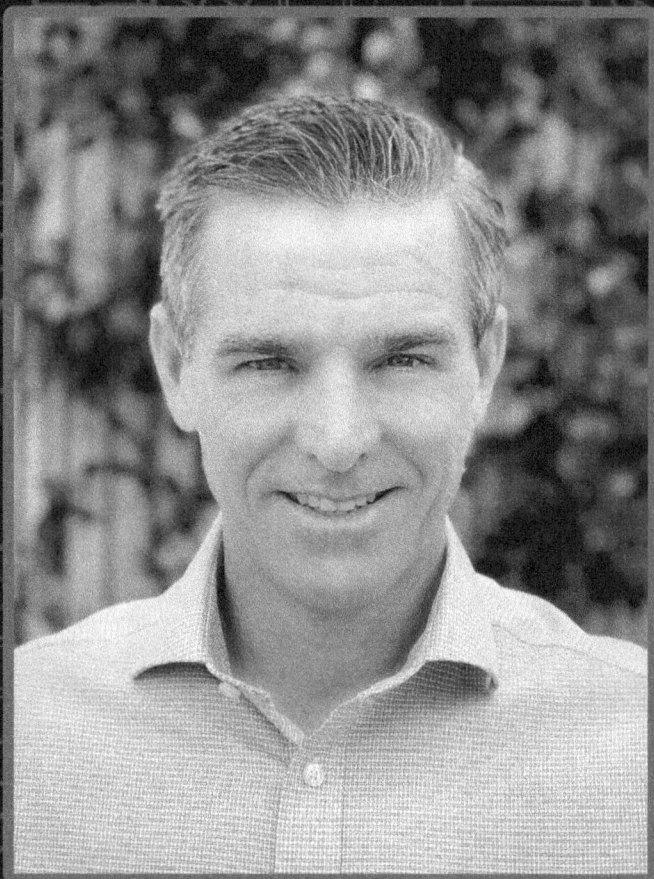
Brisbane's Mater Mothers' Hospital neonatologist Dr Luke Jardine

Dear parent,

Congratulations on the birth of your baby.
A new baby is a significant life event for you and your family. We know that having a baby in the NICU can be an incredibly stressful time; however, please still try to acknowledge and celebrate the new addition to your family.

For many families, a NICU admission is a long journey with many ups and downs (hopefully there will be more ups than downs).

The following is a list of suggestions that may help you during your stay in the NICU.

Do's

- Touch and cuddle your baby wherever possible, the staff will show you how. Skin-to-skin contact has many benefits for you and your baby.
- Talk or read to your baby.
- Ask the staff lots of questions about what and why we are doing the things we do. There is no such thing as a stupid question. Even if you have asked the question before don't be afraid to ask it again (or seek a second opinion). The staff will provide you with lots of information, and it takes a while to sink in.
- Get involved with caring for your baby (changing nappies, monitoring leads etc). If you don't know how to do it, ask the staff to show you.
- Trust your instincts – you will quickly know what your baby likes and dislikes. Parents will often be the first to identify if a baby is becoming unwell.

If you don't think your baby is acting normally, let the staff know your concerns.

- Ring us at any time if you want to check on how your baby is going.
- Read the orientation information provided.
- Learn how to wash your hands properly – the staff will show you how. Minimising the risk of infection is one of the most important things you can do.
- Take time out of the nursery to look after yourself, sleep when you can, go for a walk, etc.
- Speak to other parents about their journey. Many parents make lifelong friends from their time in the NICU.
- Express breast milk (EBM) — start as soon as possible the midwives and lactation consultants will help show you how. Breast milk has many benefits and is incredibly beneficial for preterm infants. Depending on how premature or unwell they are, they might not be able to breastfeed, but we can put it down a tube directly into their stomach. If you can't express for whatever reason, ask the staff about the possibility of using donor EBM.
- If approached about having your baby in a research study, think about it carefully. There are many things that we are still trying to learn and we often don't know the best way to do something. Evidence suggests that babies enrolled in research studies have better outcomes than babies who are not.
- Ask for help. If you are struggling, many people will be there to support you. The hospital will have access to social workers and psychologists. You can also approach family and friends (sometimes you need to give them a specific task — they want to help; however, they often don't know what to do). Your personal GP can also be a great help.

Don'ts

- Watch the monitoring equipment (I know it is hard not too) that is our job. If an alarm is sounding, try not to worry – staff will quickly attend if concerned.
- Get too focussed on the minute details. Everyone does things slightly differently. The most important thing is the end goal of having a healthy baby at the time of discharge. If you can relax and trust the staff caring for your baby (we have lots and lots of training and experience), you will find your NICU admission much easier.
- Touch any of the buttons or silence alarms (unless asked to by the staff).
- Get involved in the care of other babies. Your focus should be on your own.
- Visit if unwell with any coughs, cold-like or gastro symptoms. Wait until you are feeling better.

Admission to the NICU is an experience that will change your life forever. At the time, it feels like it will never end; however, I hope that it will be something you will be able to look back on positively in the future.

Once again, congratulations on your new arrival.

- **Brisbane's Mater Mothers' Hospital neonatologist - Dr Luke Jardine**

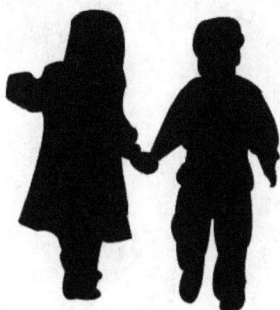

12

Preterm birth can be traumatic

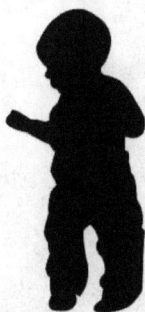

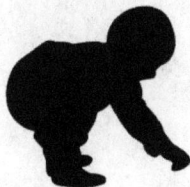

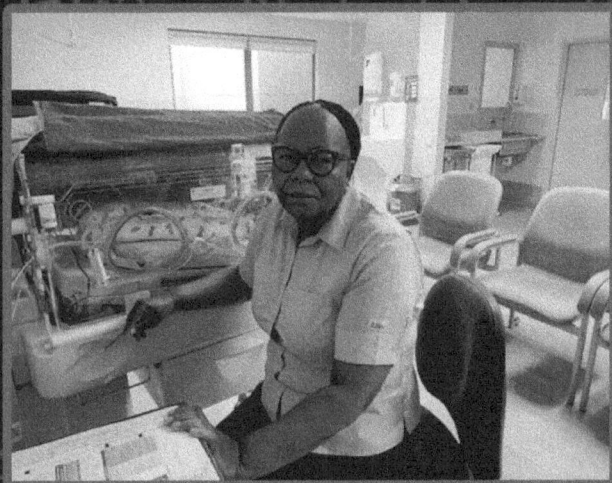
Fikile Nkwanyana, NICU nurse

Fikile Nkwanyana is a nurse with 35 years' experience. She has worked in a NICU for 23 years. Fikile is currently working at Brisbane's Mater Mothers' Hospital.

I think there's always attachment when it comes to these fragile babies. Being in NICU is such an emotional roller coaster. One always has to step back and assess the level of stress the parent might be experiencing. One thing I always endeavour to do is to show love for the baby. So when the parents can't be there, they can always have that assurance that their baby is loved and well taken care of. Preterm birth is a stressful event for families. In particular, unexpected early delivery may cause negative feelings in both parents. Preterm birth is defined by the World Health Organisation as birth that occurs before 37 weeks of gestation.

Until the nineties, prematurity was defined on the basis of birthweight, however, in recent years gestational age has been considered the main indicator of physical and neurological maturation of preterm babies. Preterm birth is a multi-problematic event that presents two main consequences. First of all, the medical and neurophysiological conditions of the newborn preterm baby put him or her in danger (particularly for infants with a weight lower than 1500g, with a gestational age lower than 32 weeks). Secondly, it could have a negative impact both on the mother and the father's relationship and on parent-child interactions. Although it has been widely demonstrated that preterm infants are at risk for developing deficits and delays, the underlying causes of these poorer outcomes and the role of parents are still less understood.

One month after preterm births, parents are shocked by the physiological and psychological conditions of their baby, and this could potentially interfere with their transition to parenthood.

The adverse medical condition of their baby prevents parents from taking care immediately of their newborn child. With their baby's prolonged stay in neonatal intensive care unit (NICU), parents usually feel powerless and helpless. This may result in parents feeling more stressed and vulnerable to emotional difficulties compared with their full term cohorts.

Preterm birth can be a traumatic event that affects parents' everyday lives. In most cases, preterm birth is the unexpected result of medical complications for the mother, which makes necessary the immediate interruption of pregnancy often in an emergency situation, to prevent serious threats to the baby's and mother's health. It could also be viewed as a traumatic event because of its threat to the physical integrity of the mother and baby. This traumatic experience has the potential of resulting in post-traumatic stress symptoms of avoidance, hyperarousal, and intrusion preventing them from having a normative transition to parenthood and damaging relationships between them and their baby.

The difficult medical conditions of premature babies and mechanical environment in NICU often prevent skin-to-skin interaction between parents and their baby — this could be dangerous for the future development of the child. Most extremely low birth weight infants will mostly spend their first 100 days of life in hospital. This extended hospital stay often exacerbates feelings of impatience, anxiety and stress.

It is therefore the responsibility of the nursing professionals to be sensitive and skilled in the use and choice of words to preserve any positive expectations at different stages of baby's clinical evolution.

Parents of premature babies often have to leave their regular routines and spend many hours in NICU where they continue to experience baby's fragility and mortality.

They live in a state of psychological and physical separation from their baby aggravated by the artificial environment of NICU. Medical staff take care of their infant's neuropsychological and behavioural development and wellbeing, which further complicates their pain and distress. The sense of powerlessness and impairment can alter the parental role, and it can also increase anxiety, depression, helplessness, frustration, guilt and anger.

In parents of preterm infants, external infant characteristics associated with immaturity and severity of medical status can be further stressors that can impair the very first relationship between the parents and their baby. The appearance of preterm babies is perceived as less attractive than features of full-term infants. They are immature and show less infantile facial features. In general, parents should try to establish a balance between adaptive or nonadaptive behaviours in order to complete a functional transition to parenthood.

Some studies have suggested that parents of premature babies are 'preterm parents' negative feelings, stress, anxiety and the uncertain future of their babies put them in a position of fragility that could damage their attachment relationship with their babies.

Therefore, supporting parents during hospitalisation of infants could prevent the development of the preterm family. Both parents are at risk after a preterm birth.

The hospital intervention approaches should focus on a family-centred approach and endeavour to improve parental involvement in the care of their infant from the beginning, allowing them part of the decision making process and ensuring that they realise they have an active role in the care of their baby.

Much of current support starts at an early stage once the diagnosis of preterm birth has been confirmed by enlisting the help of the neonatologists.

Most conversations are around preparation of parents, such as the possible complications of prematurity, answering all their questions in an attempt to alleviate undue anxiety and involving them in every decision making process at every stage of any medical interventions implemented as part of care of their premature baby.

Fortunately, medical interventions in neonatology are at such an advanced level that, despite all the stress that parents endure during their preterm baby's stay in NICU, the end reward is that most of them would still take a healthy baby home.

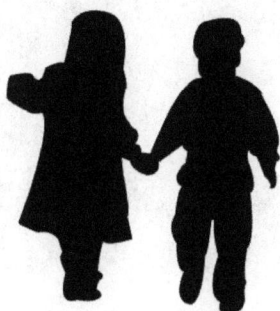

13

Losing two babies changed me

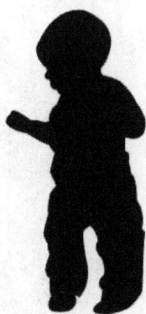

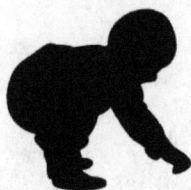

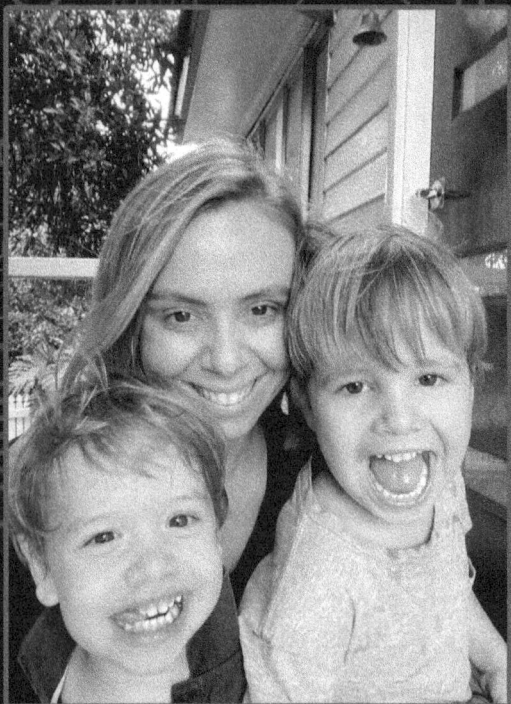
Megan with her two boys Ted and Parker.

To a fellow mum who has gone through something similar to me, I want to reassure you that you are not alone. I find it really hard to talk about what we went through because it was such a difficult time for my husband and I. I'm trying to open up more about what happened to me. In 2014 we found out I was pregnant. We reached 12 weeks' gestation and shared the news with family and friends. Everyone was really excited for us. At my 20 week scan I found out we were having a boy — more excitement. At 22.5 weeks I went into labour and gave birth to Ollie. He was alive when he was born but he couldn't be saved because he had not reached the gestational age of 25 weeks, where medical intervention could take place.

I still remember the way I felt when all of this happened. So much pain and sadness. Saying goodbye to him was the hardest thing I have ever done.

I remember holding Ollie. I visited him for the next four days at the hospital. Saying goodbye was really hard. We had a service for him with just close family. And I remember him being tall.

I fell pregnant again with another baby boy, Hugo. He only made it to 16 weeks before I lost him. This was painful, sad and I thought more than I could handle. I wasn't giving up. I really knew I was meant to be a mum and we kept trying, even with a round of IVF which failed. I eventually fell pregnant again naturally and at 20 weeks we found out it was another boy.

Through the whole pregnancy, I felt like I was holding my breath and waiting for something bad to happen.

When I reached 30 weeks I had this feeling everything was going to be okay. I gave birth to Ted in 2017, full-term. He is now three and makes me smile every day.

I gave birth to Parker (full-term) in September 2018. He is now two and the most affectionate, sweet and assertive little boy.

We have the ashes for Ollie at home and we light a candle for Ollie and Hugo every year on the day they were born. I am so lucky and blessed to have two healthy boys. I know I was meant to be a 'boy mum', as all four or my pregnancies were boys. Our family is now complete, along with our beautiful and patient rescue dog Julia.

Losing two babies changed me and I think about them every day. I hope my story helps in some way.

- Megan Cutler

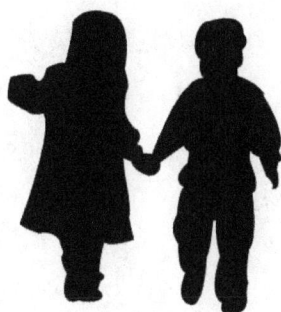

14

'She made us stronger'

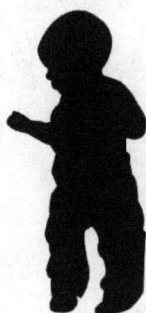

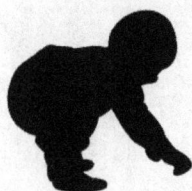

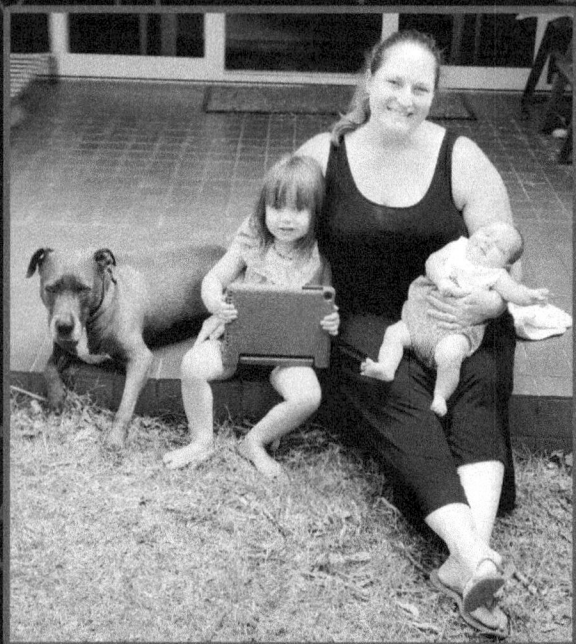
Jasmine completes the Duran family

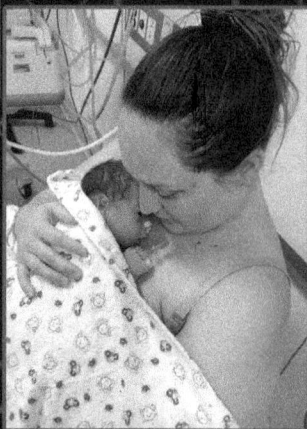
Zoe was born almost five weeks early.

Zoe Emilia, or our little FOMO (Fear Of Missing Out) baby (as my sister dubbed her) joined our clan on Friday, August 11, 2017 almost five weeks early. I hadn't finished up at work. In fact my waters broke while I was sitting at my desk talking to a co-worker. I thought I had wet myself and remember calling my husband as I moved swiftly down the hall to the bathroom with an 'I just pissed myself!' shriek down the phone.

Once I realised that my waters had broken I took myself up to the hospital. I was hooked up to the heart rate monitor, nurses came and went from my bedside, then my doctor outlined a plan on how we would keep Little Miss inside for another two weeks. Zoe was also footling breech (feet down). It wasn't until my husband, mum and dad arrived at the hospital that I took a minute to realise that this was really happening. Full of bluster, I thought with all the planning, medicine and bed rest that Zoe would arrive in a couple of weeks. Again, Zoe had other ideas.

Friday morning dawned and at 9.28am, with the urging of a full bladder, I decided to start my morning ablutions. Then I felt something.

Remember in pre-natal classes when the nurse said "if you feel something hanging where there shouldn't be anything DO NOT TOUCH IT. It may be the umbilical cord and you could damage the cord if you tug or touch it?" My (incredible, angelic) midwife happened to be in my room when I hesitantly called out "Christine, I think I feel something!" In a matter of seconds the emergency button was pushed. I was up on my bed on hands and knees and Christine was behind me pushing everything back inside.

I had something called a prolapsed cord and this required an emergency c-section.

Zoe was delivered at 9.45am. That's how quick it was. Zoe weighed 2.286kg, was 52cm long and perfect. I woke to see my husband walking towards me. I was angry. Why was he with me? Why wasn't he with my child? "Are you okay? What are we going to call her?" he asked. "Men" I responded (rather crankily). "What are you doing? Why aren't you with our child? You KNOW what we are calling her. Here, give me the pen and I'll write it down! I want to see her, I want to see Zoe," I said.

I was wheeled over to the Special Care Unit and there, in a plastic bubble, was my daughter. Relief. She was okay. She was here. Thank goodness. Our midwife, nurses, OBGYN, paediatric doctor and chaplain all told us how lucky we were that I was already in the hospital when the cord "fell out". A footling breech, and prolapsed cord birth is quite difficult, and if I had been at home or work or anywhere that wasn't a hospital, we could have potentially had a very different outcome. That scared us.

I was taken back to my room and told to rest, but how could I rest when my daughter was all the way down the hall? My husband sat with me while we called loved ones to share our news. I wanted to see Zoe and sit with her as much as I could. And tell her mummy loves her. And I'm sorry, I stuffed up. It was a strange mix of emotions, but the overwhelming feeling of love was paramount.

A week went by where we worked at bringing on my milk. Zoe was diagnosed as having jaundice, so was put under UV light for 48 hours. We slept, ate and had visitors pop in. I felt so loved when unexpected people came out of the woodwork to send us flowers, love and well wishes.

Wednesday, August 16 was horrible. It was the day I was released from hospital, but Zoe was going to be staying in for who knew how long. Driving down Coronation Drive at Milton (Brisbane) I sobbed like I hadn't sobbed in years. I walked into my house, into the nursery and felt a crushing level of failure. What sort of mum was I leaving my child? As a new mum, this should be one of the happiest days of my life, bringing my child into our home and celebrating our newest adventure. Instead, we hurriedly put together our clothes, grabbed the dog and went to stay at my parent's house for the next few weeks.

Our new norm included a pumping schedule (every two hours, night and day), getting up to go to the hospital, staying at the hospital until about 12pm, coming home to rest and then going up again in the evening so my husband could visit with Zoe. We would then go home about 7.30pm but be back again after 9.30pm to drop off the last milk for the night feeds. This is what I had to do to prove to myself I was a good mum. Every morning walking into the NICU I would search for her little head of black hair, confirm that she was okay and finally take the first proper breath of the day. It was exhausting, but I got through it with the love and support of my parents and sister, my husband and the incredible special care nurses at the hospital.

On August 30, we were told we would be staying two nights in a room WITH Zoe!!! And we were incredibly happy. We were a family. By September 1 we were finally able to bring our daughter home, just in time for my husband's first Father's Day. A new level of fear arose – why were they letting me leave with this tiny human? I'm not experienced enough to keep her, I thought to myself. But oh my goodness, it was such an amazing drive back to our house in Indooroopilly (which probably took a lot longer than was necessary).

The feeling of failure, of letting Zoe down, of guilt because my husband wasn't in the room when Zoe was delivered, of sadness that I didn't get to 'witness' Zoe's arrival, would sit with me for a very long time. I would spontaneously burst into tears whenever I thought of Zoe's birth-day and delivery. When my husband brought up having a second child, roughly around Zoe's first birthday, I started to shake: was I ready to potentially go through all of this again? I knew things in my head weren't 'right', so I booked in to see my GP to do a mental health plan. I then went and saw a psychologist who listened to my fears and my perceived failings.

Two years (and two months) on the feelings of guilt and failing from the beginning are still there, but they are overwhelmed by the feelings of love, relief, happiness, pride and thankfulness that my child is a thriving, strong, resilient, beautiful person who has changed our lives in so many positive ways.

She has made us stronger. We went through something as new parents, but we did it together and showed that the love between us was strong enough to withstand this trial.

It took me a few years but I was finally ready to have another baby. On August 27, 2020 we welcomed our second baby girl Jasmine Sophia Duran at 7.59am, weighing 3.4kg.

Leading up to our scheduled c-section date, I know I experienced a huge amount of nerves, fear of the known and unknown. After speaking with my mum I found out she was also experiencing a level of PTSD (post traumatic stress disorder) and fear which helped me recognise I needed to really look after myself and the baby, especially in the last few weeks of pregnancy.

Were we going to have the same thing happen again? Was our baby going to be okay. What would go wrong this time? This time it was perfect. This time I got to share the day with my husband. It was incredible having him there to hold my hand throughout the c-section procedure — he even got to cut the cord.

Our five days in hospital consisted of having our baby in the room with us the whole time, feeding on demand and many, many dirty nappies. On home day we went straight to my parents' house to pick up my eldest and introduce her to her baby sister Jasmine. Zoe is our miracle, while our second daughter completes our family. And we couldn't be happier.

- Meagan Duran

108

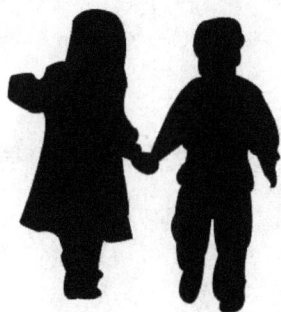

15

Lean on loved ones

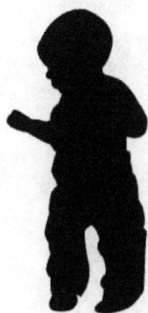

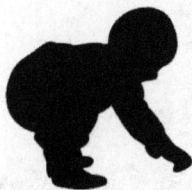

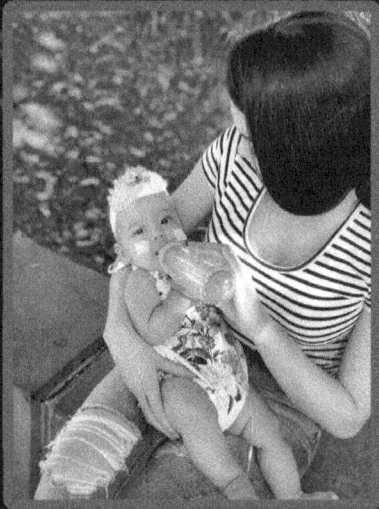

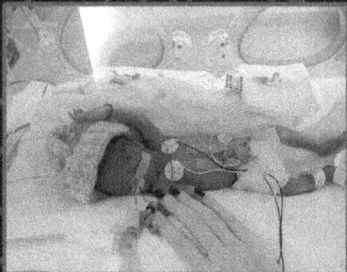

Tallulah was born at 26+1 weeks' gesta[tion],
weighing under 1kg.

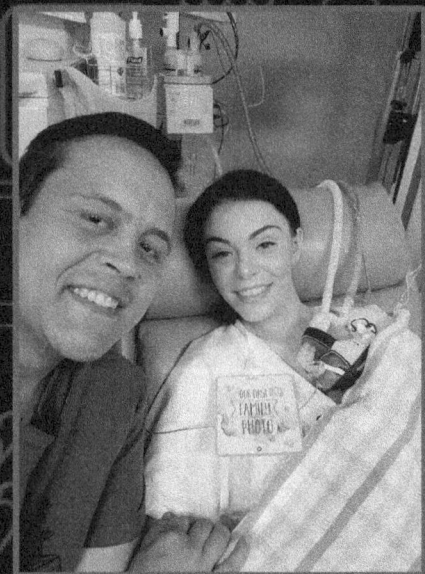

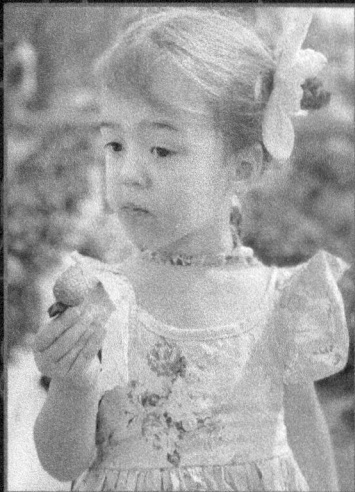

Tallulah has grown into a beautiful and happy girl and is getting ready to
welcome her baby brother to the family.

Jake and I were married in September 2016. We had waited to start our family until we had financially secured ourselves after buying our house, and did some travelling together.

Jake and I both work with children and were so excited to start our family together. We fell pregnant almost right away with a little boy. My pregnancy was a dream. The weekend before he was born we were away in Melbourne, enjoying good food, some shows, and my sister (who was also pregnant) and her partner's company. It was the first weekend I had people offer me their seats in public and I was just absolutely loving my growing baby bump.

We returned home and I went back to work. However, at 23+2 weeks' gestation, I felt some pains in my stomach at night. I thought it wasn't a big deal and tried to get to sleep. After about an hour with the pain becoming stronger, I called my local hospital. They advised me to take some Panadol and have a warm shower. If the pain did not subside in an hour, I was to come in and get checked. But when I got out of bed and prepared for my shower I noticed some spotting, and my husband and I rushed straight in. They listened to baby, and as I was not bleeding anymore they reassured me everything looked fine and I was likely going home. They just wanted to quickly check my cervix. They then told me I was 7-8cm dilated and would be having my baby that night.

Elliott was born the next morning at 7.56am, 30cm long, 20cm head circumference and weighing 566g. Our hearts were absolutely shattered, and I felt so angry with the universe. How could that have happened to our baby?

What had I done wrong? We were told there was no medical reason for losing our baby, and when we felt emotionally ready, we were able to try again but be monitored for cervical insufficiency.

I was informed I had a placental abruption, but did not have any of the typical risk factors and it was just unlucky and more than likely would not happen again.

After research and speaking with my medical team, we decided to try again to grow our family. Six weeks later, we fell pregnant again. This time I was referred to a high risk clinic and was reassured everything was totally fine. However, I was filled with anxiety. At my 18 week cervical length scan my cervix shortened under 3cm to 2.8cm. I was very distressed by this, but my 20 week scan was cancelled despite my requests to keep it.

At my 22+6 week scan it was discovered I was 2cm dilated with funnelling, and bulging membranes. It was our fear. I was immediately admitted and monitored overnight for signs of labour. The next morning I was sent down for another scan, this time 3cm dilated. I was lucky enough to not be in labour and was sent for a cervical cerclage. It was successful. It gave me 1.6cm of cervical length. The next few weeks were incredibly difficult. I was readmitted into the hospital several times, given Nifedipine to stop my labour, and also steroids for my daughter's lungs. At 25+5 weeks' gestation I experienced another bleed and was admitted to hospital.

This time it was discovered I had dilated 3cm and torn through my stitch. I did not allow them to cut it and spent the next three days in hospital with contractions and bleeding.

Then at 26+1 weeks' at 9.36am, my daughter Tallulah was born. Her eyes were open and she was crying.

She was immediately rushed off to NICU where she spent the first three months of her life. She was 30cm long, head circumference 24cm, and weighed just 940g. While she was in hospital she struggled to gain weight, and tolerate EBM (expressed breast milk).

She had a huge distended tummy and was jaundiced. At around week two her oxygen and CPAP (continuous positive airway pressure) requirements went back up. She had a grade- one bleed on her brain and anaemia of prematurity, which required three blood transfusions. She also developed stage two Retinopathy of Prematurity (ROP) which self-resolved (thank goodness). ROP is an eye disease which can happen in premature babies. It causes abnormal blood vessels to grow in the retina, and can lead to blindness.

As it got closer to Tallulah's due date, I watched the other babies in our pod come off oxygen, but my baby just didn't seem to cope without it and we were eventually sent home with oxygen tanks. While I was obviously so excited to have her home, I was devastated to be taking all that medical equipment with us. Tallulah remained on oxygen full-time for nine months, and then only at night for an additional four months.

People would often stare or ask questions in public. We were so proud of how far she had come and was (and still is) such a beautiful and happy little girl. Looking at her now, you would never know she had such a difficult start to life – she is taller than most of her peers!

As time passed our desire for another baby grew, and despite the possibility of having another extremely pre-term baby, or another loss, we decided to try again.

This time my medical team took the risks very seriously. A preventative cervical cerclage was placed at 14 weeks. I am on Progesterone, Aspirin and taking Clexane injections daily. I am currently 20 weeks along with a little boy who we have named Coah. We already love him so much. We're scared about what might be around the corner for us, but know we are doing absolutely everything we can to keep him cooking. No matter the outcome, we will love him and our lives will be better having the opportunity to love him.

So, to other mums out there, it is a hard, emotionally draining and a scary time after a loss or if you have a seriously ill baby. Be kind to yourself, lean on the people who you love and talk to them about how you're feeling. Understand your partner might cope with things differently to you and try to stay connected. Make friends with and talk with the other mums in NICU as they will be a huge support to you, and seeing a friendly face of someone who is going through a similar circumstance to you will be a huge support and distraction from the terrible fears you are most likely focused on. No matter what happens, you will get through it. Things will be okay, it will change you. But that's not a bad thing.

- **Maeve Terare**

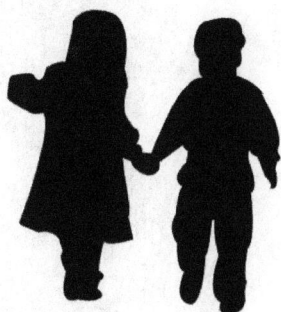

16

T21 Rocks

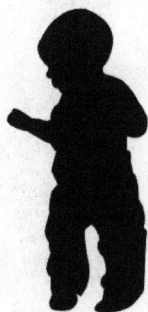

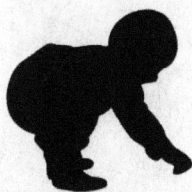

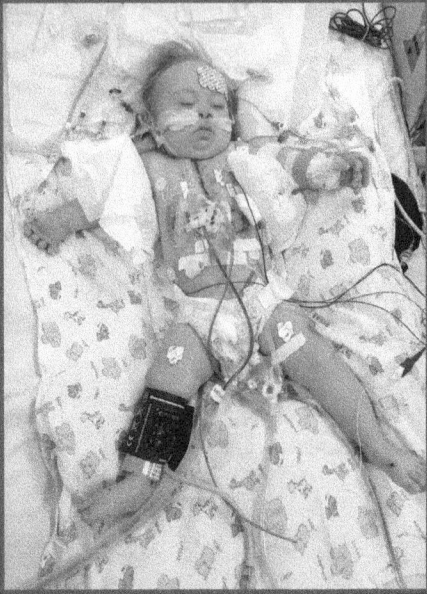

Grayson one week before his first birthday and his second open heart surgery.

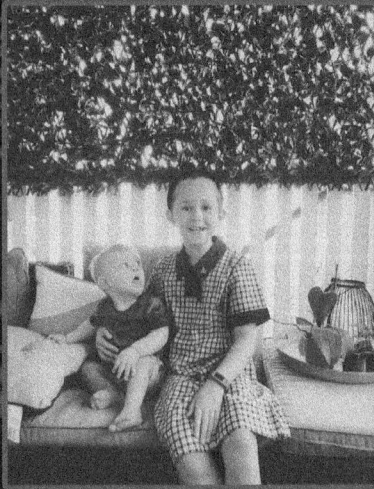

Grayson is adored by his big sister Eliette.

As if it wasn't enough to have one little miracle, we were blessed with two. In 2012, our daughter Eliette was born at 32 weeks gestation. My waters broke while in the middle of cutting my client's hair (I'm a hairdresser). There was no reason for it—I had a perfect pregnancy right up to that day.

It was a Tuesday, early evening and I had Eliette on Thursday morning at 10am. The doctor gave me medication to stop the labour, but it didn't work. I managed to have two steroid injections and I had a natural delivery. Eliette was born weighing 3 pounds 10 ounces (1.6kg). She was rushed straight to the special care nursery and thankfully could breathe on her own. I couldn't hold her until day four.

Those first few days were a blur as we navigated our new normal of humidicribs, monitors and feeding tubes. But after six long weeks, we were able to bring her home without any medical complications.

Fast forward six years later (with an ectopic pregnancy in between) our second little miracle Grayson was born. Grayson has T21 (Down syndrome) and chronic heart disease (CHD). His heart condition is quite complex. As most children born with CHD will either have one or the other, but Grayson decided that one heart condition wasn't enough. He has TOF (Tetralogy of Fallot) and AVSD (atrioventricular septal defect). He spent his first two weeks of life in NICU at Mater Mothers' before coming home for five weeks.

We were then back at the Queensland Children's Hospital after a lot of blue spells, and at eight weeks of age he underwent his first heart surgery which got him through to his major open heart surgery at just 12 months of age.

Grayson is now a mischievous two-year-old who has just started walking.

More surgeries will happen in the future for our little Grayson but for now our two little miracles are just enjoying being siblings and doing life together side by side.

I couldn't have got through the toughest of times without my husband, Luke and our little support network of family, close friends and my amazing work husband and colleagues. We had some pretty dark days, especially with Grayson when we nearly lost him six days post open heart surgery; but, we knew we needed to be strong for him and his sister.

-Julia Laine

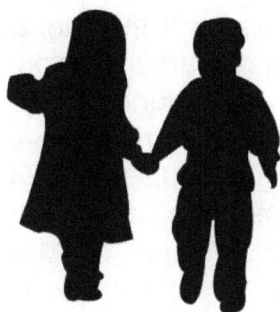

17

'I was close to dying'

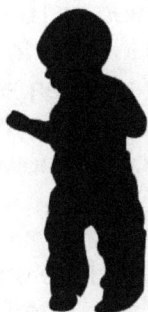

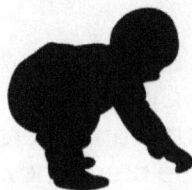

I was married at the age of 30 in 2013, and for my Indian heritage, that meant I was late to marry. My mother advised me to start a family right away, as I was now older and my response was 'I will, but after a year'. I wanted to at least enjoy a year of marriage before having a child. In 2015, my husband and I started to try but had no luck. I went to naturopaths and nutritionists. I did test after test. I took supplement after supplement. At this point, I started having a lot of period pain and went to the doctor to get medical certificates. I just couldn't go to work — it was always painful the first two days of my cycle.

In 2016, my mother suggested IVF and I thought I should do it. I did six back-to-back treatments. That was a mistake, as I didn't give my body time to recover. The whole process was mentally and physically draining. I put on a lot of weight from the fertility drugs and would constantly be told by family to lose weight.

For all treatments, I would undergo ultrasounds which showed some clusters of endometriosis and fibroids, but no one advised me to get this looked at. After each IVF treatment I lost the foetus within seven to 10 weeks. Then I did a frozen embryo transfer and lost the foetus at three months. After that I had one more frozen embryo transfer in 2018. The foetus was growing well and the heart beat was really strong. The ultrasound showed everything was growing normally.

I was so happy and I was thanking God and the universe daily. Close to five-and-a half months later I had an ultrasound and there were complications. If I proceeded with the pregnancy it would have been dangerous for my health. I had 12 hours to think about what to do.

I decided to terminate my pregnancy. I took a tablet and said goodbye to my baby. The next day I went to the hospital to complete the abortion.

I was haemorrhaging SO much I was close to dying myself. This was the most devastating time for me. I couldn't believe it. I was extremely stressed from all of it, that I started having panic attacks and would randomly start crying.

I lost hope and was so angry at the universe. I decided to see a psychologist. I stopped IVF for a year and went back to trying naturally. Still no luck. Now, it's 2020 and I'm considering IVF again. I had blood tests and ultrasounds again in March but then COVID hit – so things got delayed. From the ultrasound, the doctor strongly suggested checking my endometriosis as it could be one of the causes for my failed IVF attempts.

A surgeon was then recommended, and after meeting him I have been told there is no ultrasound machine which can really show what's happening inside — keyhole surgery is the better option. In August I underwent keyhole surgery and they found I had severe stage four endometriosis. It's all over the place – on my bowel, tubes and walls. This would explain my severe period pain and failed pregnancies. I have to now get these removed before I start IVF.

I am scared to be honest. The thought of this surgery and another round of IVF. When I look back at the last few years, I feel I went through most of it on my own. But I think being a woman, we are stronger than what we think.

My three life advices are:

1. Period pain should not be debilitating. If you are noticing it over some time and your doctor doesn't think much about it, go to a specialist and get the keyhole surgery done.

2. Freeze your eggs when you are young. It doesn't cost much to freeze them. When you have made your choice to start a family, you can fall back on them if you need them.

3. Your mind is a powerful thing — it can make you or break you. Mental stress can be overcome by seeking help from professionals or support groups. I didn't know so many people went through similar things like me until I shared my story. Prior to that, I thought it was just happening to me.

I wish everyone all the best on their journey and like me, not to give up.

-Anonymous

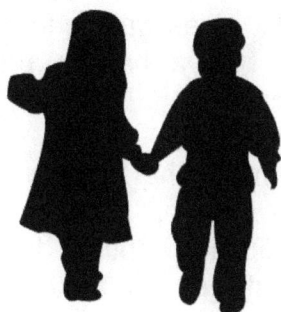

18

Waiting for my husband

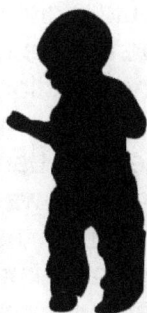

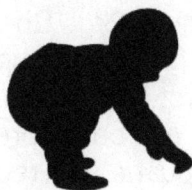

It all started when my blood pressure continued to creep up. Every night I had headaches. I contacted my obstetrician and was admitted into the hospital. I was 34 weeks + into my pregnancy. I was waiting for my baby bump to get bigger and had not yet had my pregnancy pictures taken with my husband.

My husband took me to the hospital one morning and then headed to Stradbroke Island for work. Everyday my blood pressure medication continued to increase, but my blood pressure didn't get any better. It was blood test after blood test.

On my sixth day in the hospital, my baby's heart rate decelerated on the routine CTG (Cardiotocography, a fetal and maternal monitor) and the midwife contacted my obstetrician.

'In less than 15 minutes, I was wheeled to theatre. I remember hearing the midwife telling me congrats you're going to be a mother in a few minutes. I couldn't feel happy about it. I was filled with worry and many, many uncertainties about my baby. Before I could register what was happening, I was already lying in the theatre without my husband, prepping for an emergency c-section".

With a few tugs and pulls on my abdomen, my baby was crying. At 35+1 weeks' gestation, my baby girl was born weighing 2kg. She was skinny. Even though the staff were great and supportive, this was not how I imagined my first birth experience to be, especially with my husband not being present for the birth of our first child. I was pushed to recovery and could hear many babies crying, except mine.

She was separated from me at the special care nursery to be monitored and to gain weight.

My husband took a ferry and came to the hospital thinking our baby was not going to make it. On the third day postpartum, I felt so emotional. I had the baby blues. I felt guilty, and kept blaming myself for an underweight baby. One of the hardest things to do was to get discharged without my baby.

Everyday felt like a year to me, waiting for my baby to come home. Being separated from her after I visited everyday was hard. I was tired of pumping my breastmilk day and night.

Then, the time came when her nasal gastric tube was removed and soon after she began hitting more milestones. Here we are now with our happy baby at 17 weeks plus, weighing a healthy 5.4kg. Our journey was not an easy one, but it has made us stronger and closer as a family.

So, don't give up mumma, even though the journey seems so long and tough. There will be light at the end of the tunnel. No words can describe the feeling of happiness now, and I look forward to her eating her first solids, crawling and running.

-Anonymous

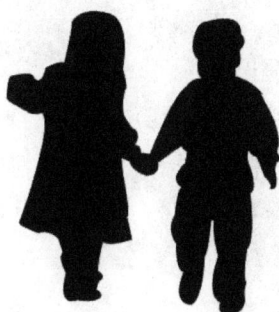

19

Breastfeeding takes practice

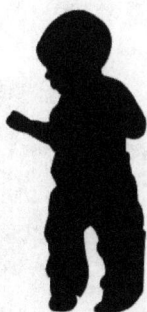

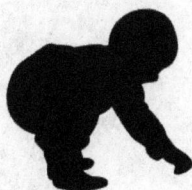

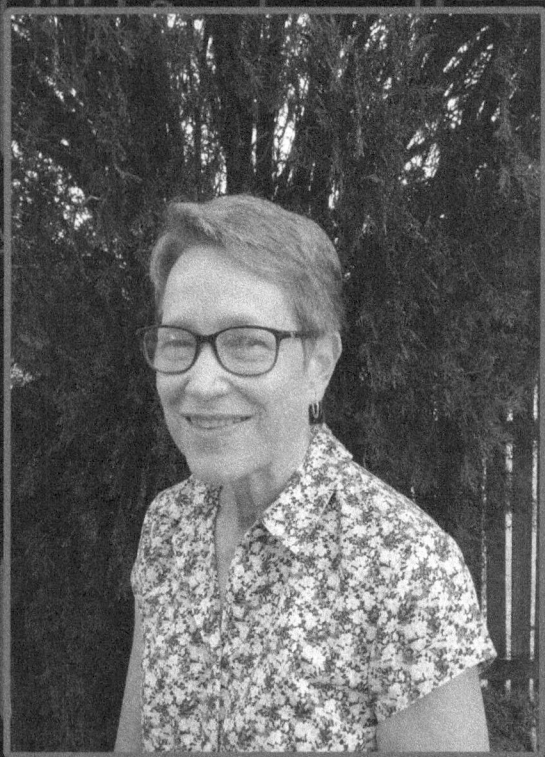
Kay Whitby, Australian Breastfeeding Association Counsellor.

Kay Whitby is a registered nurse, Australian Breastfeeding Association counsellor, and Growlife Medical Baby Clinic and Parents' Group facilitator in Brisbane.

Most parents are aware of the importance of breastfeeding for their baby's health. The lowered risk of acute infections, some chronic diseases, SIDS, obesity, malocclusion and optimising of neurological development.

Not as many are aware of the importance for the mothers' health. There is lowered risk of breast, ovarian and endometrial cancer, endometriosis, type 2 diabetes, cardiovascular disease, postpartum depression and rheumatoid arthritis. However, knowledge of this importance brings added pressure and fear of failure.

Many new mothers express anxiety about breastfeeding, worrying about the negative experiences that they may have heard. I hope I can reassure you that your baby has reflexes to come to the breast and feed.

Breastfeeding is also a learned skill that you and your little one will master over time. By reaching out for information and support you will gain confidence in your body's ability to nurture your baby at your breast. Surround yourself with a positive breastfeeding culture. Talk to your partner and family about how important breastfeeding is to you and how you would appreciate their help and support to reach your breastfeeding goals.

If you have more complex breastfeeding issues, you can be referred to an IBCLC (International Board Certified Lactation Consultant) who can be seen privately or through your maternity units' breastfeeding clinic, your local child health clinic or sometimes a breastfeeding friendly GP practice.

If you are struggling with breastfeeding, setting short-term goals may help, even if it is just getting through the next feed. For many mothers, everything falls into place after those first few weeks when breastfeeding is being established.

They are so glad they persevered through challenges, going on to love their breastfeeding relationship and the incredible bond that they experience with their baby. For many, this is a rewarding period where breastfeeding becomes quicker and easier, almost guaranteed to soothe and calm their baby and help put them to sleep.

Many mothers are able to breastfeed exclusively to the recommended around six months when solids can be slowly introduced along with continuing breastfeeding. For some mothers, breastfeeding may mean offering expressed milk, donor milk or formula as well so that their babies will grow well. This milk needs to be given in a way that protects breastfeeding. So paced bottle feeding may be suggested or a supplementary nursing system so the baby doesn't start to prefer the flow of the bottle. For some mothers, weaning support is necessary as breastfeeding is no longer working for them and their family. Sometimes they need to wean quickly or sometimes (and preferably) it can be done more slowly. Parents can be supported to bottle feed responsively and with love.

Mothers are supported through the difficult stages of breastfeeding and mothering, prematurity, twin feeding, illness, the distractible times, teething, returning to work and times when babies wake frequently.

Support is available to those who wish to breastfeed to full-term and choose to breastfeed into the second year and beyond. And support is often needed to bolster their confidence against unrealistic societal expectations of when children should wean. Please know I am here to support you, whatever your breastfeeding and parenting experience.

-Kay Whitby

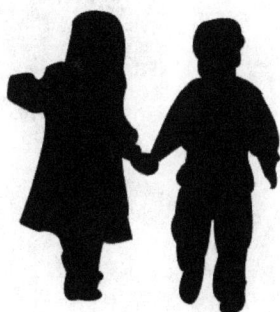

20

God has a plan

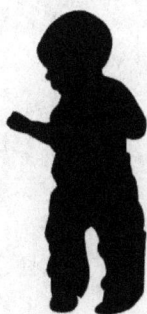

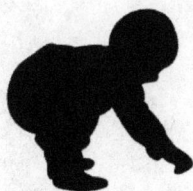

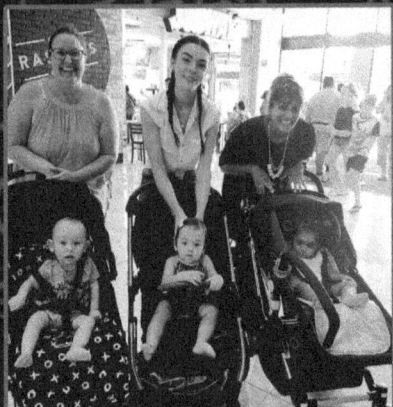
Lisa and Finn reunite with Maeve and daughter Tallulah, and Reshni and her daughter Isla.

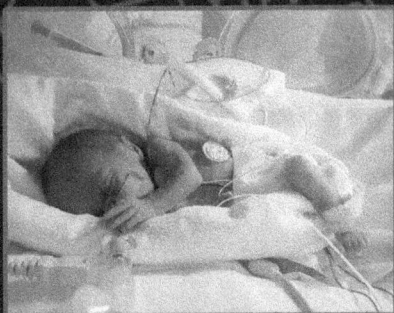
Finn in Brisbane's Mater Mothers' Hospital

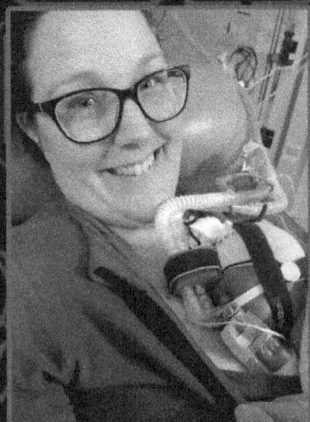
Lisa's first cuddle with baby Finn.

I started bleeding when I was nine weeks pregnant. I went to emergency and was told to expect a miscarriage. However, I had a scan and was told our baby was fine as the "heartbeat was as strong as an ox". I bled again at around 14 weeks and was told by one of the doctors that the baby would probably die. "This will not be a viable pregnancy. You will lose this baby". Another scan later and the baby was absolutely fine.

My pregnancy went along with no further problems until I had my 19 week scan. During the scan, it was noted there was a low level of amniotic fluid around my baby. My placenta was also lying extremely low as well as growing through the wall of my uterus and into my abdominal muscles. I was referred to the Mater Mothers' Hospital in Brisbane for an in-depth scan. The scan confirmed there was a low level of amniotic fluid around our baby, meaning, I needed to wait after the scan for a meeting with the head radiologist, who explained the consequences of continuing with the pregnancy whilst having such a low level of amniotic fluid.

Most of the meeting was a blur, however, certain words are ingrained into my memory. Deformed, disability, kidney failure, life support, retardation. Not words I was expecting to hear. However, they were just the beginning. As the meeting continued, the radiologist asked if I would be interested in terminating the pregnancy. At this stage, I burst into tears. Thank goodness my husband Shane was with me. I looked at him and everything in the room just blurred into a haze. I looked at Shane and said "no, I can't. I can't do this to our baby". Shane agreed. "Absolutely. We will take each day as it comes and support this baby with whatever God has planned for us," he said.

It is important to note that Shane and I were not religious people, however, as my story continues and as I relive my story, it appears that God has a plan for all of us.

The radiologist was surprised and said that should we change our minds, he could write a referral for a medical termination. "No thank you. We have made our decision", I told him. That night was a tough night and the only time I have ever heard Shane cry. At 21 weeks into my pregnancy, I remember laying in bed talking to Shane; he had just turned the light off when I felt a wetness dribble down my leg. I said "Oh no, please don't be blood again". I went to the bathroom and looked down to see clear liquid. My instinct knew this was not good. I knew it was not urine. I rang the maternity unit at my local hospital who said to come in immediately.

Shane and I raced in and I was placed on a bed. One of the doctors came in to examine me and it was confirmed. It was amniotic fluid, meaning my waters had broken at 21 weeks into my pregnancy. The next morning, I was transferred by ambulance to the Mater and admitted. That night I was visited by one of the neonatal doctors telling me that if I go into labour, our baby would die. I was also asked if I wanted the doctors to keep my baby alive if I went into labour. What a question to ask, I thought. "Um of course", I said. The doctor was surprised and reiterated that my baby would die regardless.

That night I cried myself to sleep. I was confined to bed rest at the hospital for the next week, as well as needing to take my temperature hourly and taking antibiotics. The doctors in the hospital said myself and the baby were now at risk of developing an infection.

I needed check-ups at the Mater every three days to observe my health and our baby's health as well. With all of this happening, bub was growing slowly and the weeks were passing by. "The longer he is in me, the better chance he has of surviving" I was constantly being told. I had taken leave from my job, as the doctors wanted me to rest and be close to home and to the hospital.

One Sunday morning when I was 23 weeks pregnant, I went to the bathroom. As I wiped myself, I noticed bright red blood on the toilet paper. Once again, I immediately rang the Mater and was told to get to hospital ASAP. Shane drove down and I cried most of the way not knowing what was next. I had yet another scan and once again, bub was fine and I was admitted to a room that was close to the nurse's desk. I didn't know why at this stage. I was told that I was staying in hospital now until bub was born. I had to buzz the nurse each time I went to the toilet as well as needing a catheter in my arm for my entire hospital stay. Blood needed to be taken every three days to assess my hormone levels.

Shane would visit me every few days with my boys Archie and Mitchell visiting on the weekends. My mum would also visit at the weekend as well as one of my friends. I was also visited by my team of doctors—a group of oncologists who were experts in the field of ovarian and uterine cancers. The way my placenta was growing was spreading like a cancer and due to this, I was told I needed a hysterectomy once I had bub. I was against this believing that the doctors were blowing things out of proportion. It wasn't until the doctors sat down and said to me "if you don't have a hysterectomy you will die. You will bleed out on the table and die".

I struggled mentally not being near Shane and my other children. I would cry at night missing the boys drastically and having to relay information to Shane over the phone. Week after week passed. The nurses talked of sending me home, but the doctors said no. I was okay with this, and the doctors were relieved I trusted them.

Five weeks into my stay in hospital and one Thursday night I was cramping. I was sent down to the birthing suite. They were preparing me to go into labour.

Shane was called at 11pm and told to come in. As soon as I saw him I burst into tears and he just hugged me. I was still cramping, so the nurses gave me a sleeping tablet so that I could go to sleep. I fell asleep with Shane sitting in a chair near me, quietly watching me. The cramping subsided, and I was then returned to my bed on the ward.

Shane and the boys came and visited me the next Saturday even though I was still cramping and not feeling right. They said goodbye to me that afternoon and I fell asleep before dinner time. Sunday about 5.30am, I went to the bathroom. As I wiped myself I noticed bright red blood. I buzzed the nurse. Two nurses came in by coincidence. When I told the nurses what had happened, I was surprised with what happened next. The older nurse said there was nothing to worry about as I've had bleeding in the past. The younger nurse pressed the emergency button and said "I don't care. I'm getting the doctor here". I was hooked up to the machine that monitored the baby's heartbeat. The doctor walked in, took one look at the machine and said "She's going to surgery. She needs to have this baby now".

The next bit is a blur for me. I apparently tried to ring Shane but he didn't answer. I apparently tried to ring my friend to tell her that I was having the baby and couldn't get in touch with Shane. I don't remember making these calls to this day. The next part I remember is waking up in recovery and feeling my belly. "Where's my baby?" I asked. Shane and my friend were there telling me that I had had the baby. "Is he okay?". Shane informed me our baby was in the neonatal ward hooked up on machines— alive and okay. I cried and then fell back asleep. I woke up again sometime later. Shane was there and offered me a drink. The doctors said I didn't need a hysterectomy as the placenta came away perfectly. They were just waiting to see if my blood would clot from where the placenta was removed.

About an hour later, when the doctors came to check on me, they took one look at the bag that was collecting my urine and I was raced back into surgery for an emergency hysterectomy.

Once again, I woke up in the recovery ward feeling like I'd been hit by a train. I was starting to feel more awake, however, two doctors came over to see me. "We don't know how to tell you this but after your surgery we were unable to find a clamp. We think it may be inside you. You need to go for an X-ray to determine if the clamp is in you".

After a quick x-ray, I was relieved to learn that the clamp was not in my body. It was three days until I was able to see my baby, Finn, in the neonatal ward. Shane wheeled me down in a wheelchair, right up to the humidity crib.

As soon I saw Finn, I just burst into tears. I felt such an immense feeling of guilt and failure. I felt my body had failed him and put him in this position. Shane reassured me by saying he was in a great place that would support his growth and development. It was hard to leave Finn by himself in that crib. Who would comfort him when he cried? Was that my job? Would he think I didn't love him or I don't want him?

After 10 days, my mental health deteriorated. I needed to get home to my husband, my rock and support who I had perceived in my anxiety-riddled world was distancing himself from me. Of course this wasn't true, but after the past few months of being apart, that's what I was thinking. The nurses agreed I needed to get home, however, I needed to see my GP within 48 hours for a mental health assessment. That afternoon I said goodbye to Finn crying to Shane. "He should be with me. I can't leave my baby in the hospital. It's not right", I said. I struggled with this for the next few weeks, but seeing the way in which he was growing and developing, he needed to be there.

Fast forward to December 18, 50 days after Finn was born, and I arrived at the hospital for my regular daily routine visit of breastfeeding him as soon as I arrived. The nurse came and saw me: "You're taking him home today. He's coming home with you today." I burst into tears and hugged my boy even tighter.

The past three years have had its ups and downs health-wise for Finn. Continuous doctor appointments, growth and development clinics and check-ups galore. The result of having little amniotic fluid? A boy who is absolutely healthy and who will live a full and long life.

Another result? He will always be on the tiny side. What three-year-old still fits into 00 size clothing? But hey, at least he's getting good wear out of his clothes!

- Lisa Krings

Conclusion

The aim of this book is to normalise pregnancy, birth and the challenges so many women around the world are going through every single day.

It's time to open up and talk to one another about infertility and the emotional toll IVF has on a woman and her partner. It's a waiting game from beginning to end.

Women don't often talk about miscarriage or the loss of a baby until several months after their traumatic experience.

Seeking support from loved ones and medical professionals is important.

You don't have to be rich and famous to be heard. You are human and your feelings, emotions, and wellbeing is important.

Motherhood is good, bad and sometimes ugly, we need to band together and share how we all got there, and why so many of us are still struggling.

www.ingramcontent.com/pod-product-compliance
Lightning Source LLC
Chambersburg PA
CBHW032146020426
42334CB00016B/1241